Scientific Writing and Publication Strategies for Oral Health Professionals

Rodrigo Mariño • Sergio E. Uribe
Ebingen Villavicencio-Caparó
Editors

Scientific Writing and Publication Strategies for Oral Health Professionals

Springer

Editors
Rodrigo Mariño
Melbourne Dental School
The University of Melbourne
Melbourne, Australia

Center for Research in Epidemiology, Economics and Oral Public Health (CIEESPO)
University de la Frontera
Temuco, Chile

Department of Conservative Dentistry and Oral Health
Riga Stradins University
Riga, Latvia

Monash Health Dental Services
Melbourne, Australia

Ebingen Villavicencio-Caparó
Universidad Católica de Cuenca
Cuenca, Ecuador

Universidad Peruana Cayetano Heredia
Lima, Perú

Sergio E. Uribe
Department of Conservative Dentistry and Oral Health
Riga Stradins University
Riga, Latvia

Department of Conservative Dentistry, Periodontology and Digital Dentistry
LMU University Hospital
LMU Munich, Germany

ISBN 978-3-031-97915-6 ISBN 978-3-031-97916-3 (eBook)
https://doi.org/10.1007/978-3-031-97916-3

This Springer imprint is published by the registered company Springer Nature Switzerland AG
The registered company address is: Gewerbestrasse 11, 6330 Cham, Switzerland

Foreword

Oral health is at a new crossroads. After years of neglect and absence at national and global levels of decision-making, an aspiration toward better systems to prevent and treat oral diseases, reduce inequities, and improve the quality of life throughout the lifespan is experiencing thriving, encouraging events. The inflection point was the 2021 World Health Organization Resolution, which included oral health in the Non-Communicable Disease and Primary Care Agendas.

A key contributor to these developments has been the availability of scientific evidence supporting policies, objectives, and interventions. Such evidence has benefited from consequential research thinking, implementation, and dissemination. It is imperative, therefore, that the highest scientific rigor, intellectual discourse, and unbiased interpretation of findings be at the forefront of this spring in oral health. We all benefit from well-thought-out research questions, thorough methodological approaches, and timely publication of findings.

The book *Scientific Writing and Publication Strategies for Oral Health Professionals* is essential precisely because it fosters the dissemination of critical scientific findings. This manual presents and describes strategies for research writing and publication processes. Its comprehensive approach, blending theory with practical application, positions it as an indispensable resource for various stakeholders, including motivated professionals, research scholars, faculty members, and students on their academic journeys. Furthermore, this manual aims to enhance the visibility and impact of research in oral health and beyond.

The book presents concepts and processes crucial for effective communication within the academic community through its chapters. It discusses various methods of organizing scientific writing. It covers different categories of scientific publications, including research protocols, grant proposals, manuscripts, and conference presentations, each possessing its unique format and set of expectations. By exploring these varied forms, the book aims to equip researchers with the knowledge necessary to produce impactful and well-structured publications.

The book also provides insights into bibliometrics, publication ethics, and the principles of open science, emphasizing the importance of transparency, accessibility, and reproducibility in scientific work. Guidelines and tools are included to help researchers navigate these critical aspects, ensuring that their contributions are easily accessible to peers and the public.

Chapters 6–9 offer detailed information on the essential elements of a scientific article, such as the introduction, methodology, results, and discussion. Additionally, other chapters guide researchers in selecting appropriate journals for submission, creating compelling conference materials, and navigating the intricacies of the peer-review process. Understanding the expectations and norms of publication can greatly enhance the chances of successful dissemination.

The publishing process is often complicated by various events and circumstances that can influence the timeline and effectiveness of communication. The process consists of several stages before publication, including manuscript preparation, submission, peer review, revision, and final acceptance. It is often a lengthy and sometimes frustrating process that demands significant time, effort, and resources from researchers.

The authors have organized the book to guide readers through the intricacies of scientific writing and publication, demystifying the complexities of the process while providing practical tools and strategies to facilitate successful outcomes. By understanding and mastering the steps involved, researchers can enhance their ability to share their discoveries with the broader scientific community, ultimately advancing knowledge and innovation within their fields.

Co-Director, WHO Collaborating Centre
New York University
New York, NY, USA
November 2024
Eugenio Beltrán-Aguilar

Preface

In an era characterized by rapid technological advancements and an ever-evolving scientific landscape, the methodologies and frameworks surrounding academic publishing have undergone profound transformations. The recent global pandemic has cemented a shift in academic publishing. As researchers and practitioners deal with the implications of this new normal, the need for up-to-date resources becomes increasingly apparent. *Scientific Writing and Publication Strategies for Oral Health Professionals* emerges as a timely response, providing an essential tool to navigate the complexities of modern scientific communication.

This book highlights the necessity for a comprehensive resource tailored specifically for oral health professionals while also acknowledging its broader relevance to the health sciences community. The traditional paradigms of academic publishing, long dominated by subscription-based journals and conventional publication practices, have been disrupted by the rise of open-access models. Open science, a movement advocating for transparency and accessibility in research, is gaining momentum, promoting the dissemination of scholarly outputs beyond traditional articles to include research protocols, datasets, and various innovative formats. This shift not only increases access to scientific knowledge, but also encourages collaboration and reproducibility, essential components of research. However, despite the advantages of this new paradigm, new challenges are posed by predatory journals and the evolving metrics used to assess research impact.

While the primary focus is on oral health professionals, the insights and strategies presented are relevant to a diverse audience, encompassing undergraduate and postgraduate students, as well as health professionals seeking to enhance their scientific writing skills. The Manual seeks to provide an in-depth exploration of the "what" and "why" of open science, as well as practical strategies for navigating the contemporary publishing landscape. By exploring the complexities of scientific writing, this manual aims to equip readers with the necessary skills to effectively communicate their research findings for public consumption.

In addition to addressing the technical aspects of writing and publication, the manual also emphasizes the importance of ethical considerations in scientific communication. The rise of predatory journals, which exploit the open-access model for profit rather than for the advancement of knowledge, poses a significant challenge to the integrity of academic publishing. This book equips readers with the tools to recognize and avoid such pitfalls, ensuring that their work is published in reputable journals that uphold rigorous peer-review standards.

The authors expect that *Scientific Writing and Publication Strategies for Oral Health Professionals* addresses the pressing needs of today's researchers in a rapidly changing academic publishing environment. By providing an exploration of open science, ethical publishing practices, and effective communication strategies, this manual empowers oral health professionals and health sciences professionals in general to navigate the complexities of scientific publishing with confidence and competence.

Melbourne, Australia — Rodrigo Mariño
Riga, Latvia — Sergio E. Uribe
Cuenca, Ecuador — Ebingen Villavicencio-Caparó

Contents

About the Editors and Contributors

About the Editors

Rodrigo Mariño, CD, MPH, PhD is a public health dentist and professorial fellow at the Melbourne Dental School, The University of Melbourne, Australia, where he has worked since 2004. Prof. Mariño has a dental degree from the University of Chile, a master's in public health (University of Minnesota), and a PhD from the University of Melbourne. He also has an Honorary appointment with the Faculty of Dentistry, Universidad de la Frontera in Temuco, Chile, and holds a position at the Population Oral Health and Research, Dental Services Monash Health in Melbourne, Australia, and at Riga Stradins University, Latvia. He has also been a consultant to the Pan American Health Organization/World Health Organization in Washington, DC.

Prof. Mariño's research focuses strongly on oral health promotion and reducing inequalities in oral health status. He has excellent research expertise in social epidemiology, health economics, dental workforce issues, public health, migrant health, information and communication technology, gerontology, and population oral health. He has established links and maintains continuous contact and research activities with major research and academic groups in Australia and overseas. He has published more than 190 papers in scientific journals, several major research reports, 50 book chapters, and 5 books.

Prof. Mariño was a founder and first President of the e-Oral Health Research Network, International Association for Dental Research (IADR), and serves on the Editorial Boards of the *Journal of Dental Research*, *BMC Oral Health*, *Dental Traumatology*, and *Gerodontology*.

Sergio E. Uribe, DDS, MSc, PhD is an Associate Professor at the Department of Conservative Dentistry and Oral Health, Riga Stradins University, Riga, Latvia, and Visiting Professor at LMU Klinikum, LMU, Munich, Germany. He holds a DDS, is a Specialist in Maxillofacial Radiology (MSc), and has a PhD. Prof. Uribe's research interests include diagnostic imaging, cariology, artificial intelligence, meta-research, and dental education. He is the Principal Investigator of the Global Initiative on AI for Health (GI-AI4H), a collaborative effort by WHO/ITU/WIPO to advance the application of artificial intelligence in dentistry. Prof. Uribe serves on the editorial boards of the Journal of Dental Research and the Dental Traumatology Journal and has reviewed over 400 papers for more than 30 journals. In 2007, the International Dental Association in New Orleans, USA, honored him with the Research in Prevention Travel Award.

Ebingen Villavicencio-Caparó, CD, Esp., Mg., PhD, is a dental surgeon with a master's degree in Stomatology from the Peruvian University Cayetano Heredia, a doctorate in Health Sciences from the Catholic University of Santa María, Arequipa, Peru. Prof. Villavicencio is a specialist in Statistics and a researcher accredited by the National Secretariat of Science and Technology SENESCYT of Ecuador. He works as a professor of scientific writing and research methodology in postgraduate courses in Ecuador, Peru, and Bolivia. He was appointed as a member of the committee of experts in oral health of the Ministry of Health of Peru. He was responsible for the publications of journals and books at the Catholic University of Cuenca, Ecuador. He was also Chief Editor of the EDUNICA Catholic University Editorial of Cuenca, Ecuador. He has contributed to publications of journal articles and books on oral health epidemiology and philosophy of science. He was academic coordinator of the doctorate in Stomatology at the Universidad Peruana Cayetano Heredia and is currently a professor of statistics and philosophy of science in the same doctorate. He is currently the academic coordinator of the master's degree in public health at the Catholic University of Cuenca, Ecuador.

Contributors

Amalia Kermond-Mariño Department of Anatomy and Physiology, The University of Melbourne, Melbourne, VIC, Australia

Maura Klenner Departamento de Lenguas, Literatura y Comunicación, Universidad de la Frontera, Temuco, Chile

Rodrigo Mariño Melbourne Dental School, The University of Melbourne, Melbourne, Australia

Center for Research in Epidemiology, Economics and Oral Public Health (CIEESPO), University de la Frontera, Temuco, Chile

Department of Conservative Dentistry and Oral Health, Riga Stradins University, Riga, Latvia

Monash Health Dental Services, Dandenong, Melbourne, VIC, Australia

Estefanía Patiño-Ramon Universidad Católica de Cuenca, Cuenca, Ecuador

Sergio E. Uribe Department of Conservative Dentistry and Oral Health, Riga Stradins University, Riga, Latvia

Department of Conservative Dentistry, Periodontology and Digital Dentistry, LMU University Hospital, LMU Munich, Germany

Ebingen Villavicencio-Caparó Universidad Católica de Cuenca, Cuenca, Ecuador

Universidad Peruana Cayetano Heredia, Lima, Perú

List of Abbreviations

AAS	Asian Academic Society
AJOL	African Journals Online
ANID	Agencia Nacional de Investigación y Desarrollo
APA	American Psychology Association
APC	Article processing charges
BASE	Bielefeld Academic Search Engine
BMC	BioMed Central
BMJ	British Medical Journal
CoCoPop	Condition, context, population
CONSORT	Consolidated Standards of Reporting Trials
CORE	COnnecting REpositories
CPI	Community Periodontal Index
CPI	Consumer Price Index
CSV	Comma-separated values
DECS	Health descriptors
DMF	Decay, missing, and filled index
DMP	Data management plan
DOAJ	Directory of Open Access Journals
DOI	Digital object identifiers
DORA	Declaration on research assessment
ECLIPSe	Expectations, Client group, Location, Impact, Professionals, Service
EQUATOR	Enhancing the QUAlity and Transparency Of health Research
ERC	European Research Council
ERIC	Education Resources Information Center
FAIR	Findable, accessible, interoperable, and reusable
FINER	Feasible, interesting, novel, ethical, and relevant
HTML	Hypertext markup language
IMRaD	Introduction, methods, results, and discussion
ISBN	International Standard Book Number
ISRCTN	International Clinical Trials Registry Platform
ISSN	International Standard Serial Number

JSON	JavaScript object notation
J-STAGE	Japan Science and Technology Information Aggregator, Electronic
Lilacs	Latin American and Caribbean Health Sciences Literature
MESH	Medical subject heading
MLA	Modern Language Association
NGO	Non-governmental organization
NH&MRC	National Health and Medical Research Council
NIH	National Institutes of Health
OHIP	Oral Health Impact Profile
ORCID	Open researcher and contributor ID
OSF	Open Science Foundation
PDF	Portable document format
PECO	Population, exposure, comparison, outcomes
PICO	Population, intervention, comparison, outcome
PIRDS	Population, index test, reference test, diagnosis of interest
PRISMA	Preferred reporting items for systematic review and meta-analysis protocols
PROSPERO	Prospective Register of Systematic Reviews
PscyINFO	Database of abstracts of literature in the field of psychology
Redalyc	Red de Revistas Científicas de América Latina y el Caribe, España y Portugal
SciELO	Scientific Electronic Library Online
SENESCYT	Secretaria Nacional de Ciencia y Tecnologia
SMART	Specific, measurable, achievable, relevant, and time
SPIRIT	Special purpose integrated remote intelligence terminal
STARD	Standards for Reporting Diagnostic Accuracy
STROBE	Strengthening the reporting of observational studies in epidemiology
TIDieR	Template for intervention description and replication
UKRI	UK Research and Innovation
UNESCO	United Nations Educational, Scientific and Cultural Organization
URL	Uniform resource locator
WHO	World Health Organization
WoS	Web of science

List of Figures

List of Boxes

List of Tables

Chapter 1
Introduction to Scientific Writing

Rodrigo Mariño

1.1 Introduction

Scientific activity is the process of collecting, interpreting, and documenting information, developing and organizing ideas and conclusions, and communicating them in a clear manner. Scientific communication makes it possible for the knowledge acquired through research to be evaluated by peers, circulated, and made available for public consumption. This process also serves as a means for society to evaluate. This form of communication is one of the most rewarding experiences in professional work. Moreover, there is also an ethical requirement to publish the results of research.

This manual is aimed at those who wish to acquire the necessary skills to write scientific articles. It is intended for academics, undergraduate and graduate students, healthcare professionals, veditors of scientific journals in the healthcare field, supervisors of graduate projects, and academics with an interest in publishing research results in high-impact scientific journals. The manual focuses specifically on oral health professionals, but its content is relevant to all of healthcare.

Through this manual, the reader will acquire the knowledge, skills, and competencies to communicate the results of scientific research accurately, effectively, and clearly. This manual will also provide practical tips to identify how and where to

R. Mariño (✉)
Melbourne Dental School, The University of Melbourne, Melbourne, Australia

Center for Research in Epidemiology, Economics and Oral Public Health (CIEESPO), University de la Frontera, Temuco, Chile

Department of Conservative Dentistry and Oral Health, Riga Stradins University, Riga, Latvia

Monash Health Dental Services, Melbourne, Australia
e-mail: r.marino@unimelb.edu.au

R. Mariño et al. (eds.), *Scientific Writing and Publication Strategies for Oral Health Professionals*, https://doi.org/10.1007/978-3-031-97916-3_1

publish a variety of formats (poster, manuscript, reports, etc.), including submission for peer review and responding to reviewers' criticisms and comments.

The idea for this manual arises from our observation that many research experiences in dentistry remain as such: experiences that are not published or are published as a postgraduate thesis or research reports, without reaching a wider audience. However, in many cases these experiences contain valuable information and collected data that deserves to be disseminated. This was one of the main motivations for this manual, to turn these experiences into widely accessible publications.

Now, why does this happen? This is not something specific to the dentistry, in general many works remain as final reports or as a thesis, rather than a mass publication of the article. This happens for various reasons.

1.1.1 Why Do We Write?

For intellectual stimulation. As already mentioned, it is one of the most rewarding experiences for a researcher. We also write because we want to:

- Share our experiences, the ideas we have.
- Share the results of a research.
- Express our opinions on a matter.
- Generate discussion on a topic.
- Advance a discipline with research results.
- Position ourselves as experts in an area.
- Contribute to our reputation as researchers or as professionals.
- Disseminate a topic that we find interesting.
- Document the originality of our ideas.

Maybe we write because we want to immortalize ourselves and because we are after certain economic benefits. However, in general, publications are not free for the authors who write them. Sometimes, there is a cost in the publication, but this is something else that we will discuss in this manual. But in terms of economic remuneration, there is no direct financial return for the time invested.

However, there are indirect economic benefits in the sense of obtaining an academic promotion. As such, we also write because it is often a requirement to obtain academic promotions or obtain what is called a property position for which you must produce a record of publications.

Enrique Lihn was a Chilean poet, perhaps not as well-known as Pablo Neruda or Gabriela Mistral, but recognized among Chilean poets and within the region. He has a poem, and a book, called *Because I Wrote* [1]. Apart from the issue of writing, it portrays the human situation in Chile very well, but also in the rest of Latin America. However, it also speaks to us about humility in writing and as a way of loving one's neighbour. Writing is not only an intellectual activity, but it is also an act of generosity and recognition towards others. Therefore, we write with the desire to give back to the community with our achievements and knowledge, sharing what we have learned and achieved for the benefit of all. In this way, our writing becomes a bridge that unites our work with collective well-being, reflecting our commitment and gratitude to those around us.

1.1.2 Why Do We Not Write?

Now, why don't we write? This is what we want to reverse with this manual. One reason is a lack of motivation to disseminate the results of our research work. According to Jenkins and collaborators (1998), the lack of motivation to disseminate research results is due to [2]:

- Lack of interest (or time)
- Lack of confidence in the quality of one's own work. This is common in novice instigators and early career researchers. They often do not believe in the validity of their own results or have little confidence that the product of their research will be accepted by the scientific community.
  I tell these researchers that they should always feel proud of their work, because every step they take in their research is an advance and every discovery, no matter how small, contributes to collective knowledge.
- Lack of critical mass and support from mentors or peers for those who are beginning in the process of disseminating their scientific work. The absence of a support network may discourage new researchers from publishing their findings.
- Lack of skills in writing a research article. This is an ability that is learned. Scientific articles have a whole structure and process, and there are certain phrases and words that are commonly used in publications. We can learn this from our mentors, but can also be self-taught.
- Lack of a culture of research and publication of research results. This lack of research culture translates into fewer incentives and opportunities for researchers to publish their work, perpetuating a cycle of low visibility and less recognition of local research.

Research is a process of continuous learning and growth, and the value of your work should not be underestimated. Confidence in your abilities and the potential impact of your discoveries is essential for professional development. Therefore, I encourage all novice researchers to celebrate their achievements and present their results with pride. Acceptance and recognition of work will come as a result of dedication and constant effort, but it begins with confidence in the value and worth of your work.

Returning to the issue of lack of confidence in the quality of one's work, this was raised as an issue for novice researchers, but it is present for all researchers, even more experienced ones. There may always be doubt about the quality of the work. This is because researchers eventually realize that they know very little and this leads them to doubt, in their work, because they realize, as Karl Popper said, that

"*Our knowledge can only be finite, while our ignorance must necessarily be infinite*", perhaps reflecting a feeling that comes to us from ancient Greece, when Socrates said: "*I only know that I know nothing (and I am not even sure of that)*".

Maybe you have experienced it yourself. It is that feeling of being an imposter [3]. The "imposter syndrome" is a behavioural phenomenon described as doubts regarding intellect, abilities, or achievements among high-achieving people [3]. They feel like impostors, who at any moment are going to be caught as such. It is for this precise reason that we always question our work. It is not that we are impostors, but because as researchers we are continuously questioning the quality of our work because we feel that it is always incomplete.

To reverse the causes of why we do not write, it is essential to foster environments that encourage collaboration and training in scientific writing and the establishment of support systems that promote and value the publication of results.

However, as mentioned, the publication of research results is also an ethical issue. When you prepare a proposal for an Ethics Committee (see Chap. 2), there is a section which asks how the research results will be disseminated. Moreover, in order to seek funding for research, organizations will ask you about your plan for dissemination of the results. It is even possible that these organizations require specific and detailed information about previous publications, such as copies of final research reports or lists of publications resulting from completed research projects.

Therefore, it is not only a matter of ethics that obliges us to publish, but it also happens that if we want to advance in our field, we are going to need a track record of the publications that have resulted from our scientific work and those publications will be evaluated not only in terms of the works themselves, but also in terms of the impact they have had. This impact relates to how many times the publication has been cited. We will discuss this in Chap. 3.

Leonardo's quote: "*The most useful science is that whose fruit is the most communicable*" relates to this manual, as it tells us that there is a conflict between the usefulness of scientific work and its communication, present even in ancient times. This is what we are going to try to disclose in this manual. As mentioned, to write scientifically you can be self-taught, but it is also something that can be learned.

As an anecdote, I can tell you that years ago when I was starting my career, I sent my first manuscript to a high-impact scientific journal, and as you would expect, it was rejected. However, along with the rejection letter, I received a copy of a book on how to write scientific papers. I am not sure what message they were trying to convey, but clearly it was an invitation to improve my writing skills and to strive and persevere on the path of scientific research communication, knowing that constructive criticism is a fundamental part of the learning process and professional growth.

An invitation to move forward and strive to perfect our work is what we want to achieve with this manual. The emphasis will be on providing practical solutions to real problems and situations. The manual is organized into 13 chapters. The research process consists of different phases, however, in this manual emphasis will be placed on the last stage: how to present the results of an investigation and how to disseminate them, which is not a straightforward process since it is often drawn out by several events and situations. The publishing process also consists of a series of stages before reaching publication. It is a long and frustrating process, which demands time and resources.

In the following chapters, key aspects are addressed such as the document structure, clarity in the communication of results, and the correct citation of sources. It is hoped that by mastering these skills, readers will be better prepared and equipped to produce a variety of scientific documents, each tailored to a specific purpose and audience. However, the primary objective of this manual is to increase scientific production in dentistry and guide researchers in the process of submitting work for peer review in academic journals and presentation at scientific conferences.

It is our intention that this manual will act as a general guide to direct researchers on how to prepare publications, ensuring that research communication and dissemination objectives are achieved effectively for each specific audience. Our intention is for both novice and experienced researchers to improve the quality of their publications, thereby contributing to effective and professional scientific communication and, most importantly, to the advancement of knowledge.

References

1. Lihn E. Porque escribí: Antología poética. 3rd ed. Santiago de Chile: Fondo de Cultura Económica Chile, Colección TIERRA FIRME; 1995.
2. Jenkins S, Price C, Strater L. Writing a research proposal. In: The researching therapist. Churchill Livingston; 1998. p. 27–36.
3. Huecker M, Shreffler J, McKeny P, et al. Imposter Phenomenon. StatPearls; 2024.

Chapter 2
Document Taxonomy: Research Protocol, Grant Proposal, Manuscript, Conference Presentations

Rodrigo Mariño and Amalia Kermond-Mariño

2.1 General Research Considerations

2.1.1 What Is Research?

The Oxford dictionary defines "research" as "the study of materials and sources in order to establish facts and reach new conclusions" [1]. Research has also been defined as:

> a series of stages and steps that allow researchers to move from formulating a question to its answer [2].

Other definitions tell us that research is a systematic way of generating knowledge:

> a systematic process of collecting, analysing and interpreting information (data) to increase our understanding of a phenomenon that interests or concerns us [3].
>
> A systematic and principled way of obtaining evidence for solving (health care) problems and investigating (health) issues [4].

R. Mariño (✉)
Melbourne Dental School, The University of Melbourne, Melbourne, Australia

Center for Research in Epidemiology, Economics and Oral Public Health (CIEESPO), University de la Frontera, Temuco, Chile

Department of Conservative Dentistry and Oral Health, Riga Stradins University, Riga, Latvia

Monash Health Dental Services, Melbourne, Australia
e-mail: r.marino@unimelb.edu.au

A. Kermond-Mariño
Department of Anatomy and Physiology, The University of Melbourne, Melbourne, VIC, Australia
e-mail: a.kermondmarino@unimelb.edu.au

R. Mariño et al. (eds.), *Scientific Writing and Publication Strategies for Oral Health Professionals*, https://doi.org/10.1007/978-3-031-97916-3_2

Research provides us with tools to explore the world around us. It is a systematic reasoning process used to confirm existing knowledge and construct new knowledge [2].

The research process has several stages, from conceptualizing an original idea and formulating our research question, the design of the study and its conduction, to the analysis of the data, conclusions, and final recommendations. This research process refers to the continuous and iterative nature of conducting research, where each of these steps (from formulating a research question, collecting data, analyzing findings, and drawing conclusions) leads to the next, creating a cyclical process. Each of these steps must be followed rigorously. This is because if one of them is not conducted meticulously, the entire research process is at risk, and therefore the quality of the research will not meet standards. The contribution to existing knowledge will be minimal or even non-existent. A schematic of this process is shown in Fig. 2.1.

However, once we find the answer to our initial question, new questions appear that must be answered following the same process. I must emphasize this; no research and no knowledge are final, there will always be biases and limitations that force the cycle to continue. The answer to the initial question always generates more questions, that is, the cycle continues. Each answer obtained not only solves an unknown but also opens the door to new areas of exploration. This perpetual cycle is what drives the advancement of knowledge and understanding in any field. It is a reminder that human knowledge is always partial, imperfect, and constantly evolving.

In summary, scientific activity is a process of collecting, interpreting, and documenting information, developing, organizing ideas and conclusions, and communicating them clearly, which is one of the most rewarding experiences of professional work. The research process consists of different phases, however in this book we will focus on the last phase of the research process: the dissemination of the results.

2.1.2 Why Investigate?

The dream of reaching more advanced states of social and economic development can only be achieved through research. Research makes us an integral part of this process. By engaging in research, we are not only contributing to the advancement of our own discipline, but we are also actively participating in building a more promising future for our nations and strengthening their ability to compete in an increasingly interconnected world.

Research constitutes a fundamental tool for development and progress. Through the generation of new knowledge, innovation, and the resolution of complex problems, research contributes to improving people's quality of life, boosting economic growth and promoting social well-being. Furthermore, research is a key driver for sustainable development.

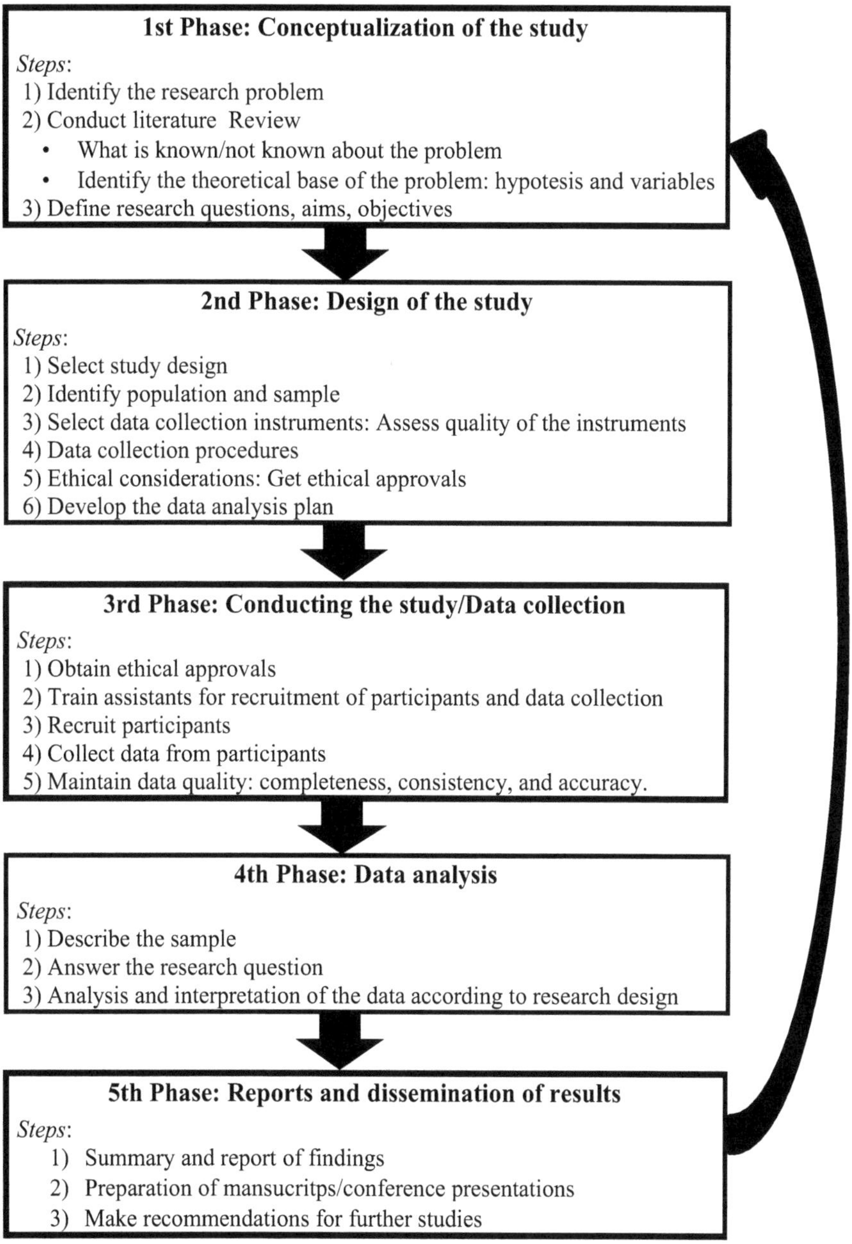

Fig. 2.1 The research process [2] (Used with permission of Elsevier, from Navigating the maze of nursing research: an interactive learning adventure, Borbasi et al., 2004 [2]; permission conveyed through Copyright Clearance Center, Inc.)

We also investigate because human knowledge is imperfect, incomplete, temporary, and subject to revision based on new evidence, theories, or interpretations; therefore, we will never reach a point where all the questions have been answered. There will always be uncertainties or gaps in human knowledge.

For these reasons, it is essential to promote a local research culture, supporting researchers at all levels of development, and promoting collaboration between academic institutions, the public and private sectors, and society in general.

2.1.3 *Where to Start?*

The process begins with an idea. All research starts from an idea, something that catches our attention, something that we think should be tried, something that is worth asking. This research idea will not emerge by spontaneous generation. The sources can be varied. For example, the question we wish to answer to may come from our own experience or clinical practice, from reading the literature, or from attending conferences and listening to what other peers or authorities in the field tell us about areas not explored in the literature or where evidence is lacking, weak, or contradictory. Discussing the topic with colleagues and/or other experts, attending conferences, where experts from different areas of dentistry gather to talk and share experiences, can all result in new research.

Apart from those or from a critical review of the literature, additional sources may be:

- Priorities of organizations that fund studies (for example, the national or regional research fund). For example, SENESCYT in Ecuador or ANID in Chile, NH&MRC in Australia, NIH in the United States.
- Priorities established by a professional discipline
- Areas of interest of professional/academic experts
- Areas of interest in a specific sector, a study center (e.g., University), a business, etc.

However, whatever the origin of that idea, this must be an area that interests us, an area that will keep us interested/passionate, given that the process is long and arduous. That passion is what will help us stay focused on the topic when resources are lacking, and when we face other obstacles during the research and publication process. This research topic or idea may be work related, however, this is not compulsory.

Furthermore, the idea to be investigated must show some tangible and relevant benefit. Funding organizations and ethics committees will be interested in how these results will not only expand theoretical knowledge, but also in how they will benefit the community and the field of study in general. These organizations want to ensure that the resources provided will contribute significantly to the advancement of knowledge, the improvement of current practices, and the well-being of people affected by the research topic. In addition, they seek to ensure that the project has a positive and sustainable impact, and that the findings can be applied in a practical way to solve real problems.

When you have selected your potential research topic, that is, when you have narrowed down your list to a single topic, do a preliminary review of the literature and answer the questions:

1. Has it been done before?
2. Is it viable?
3. Do I have the required experience and skills?
4. Do I have the time and/or the necessary resources (human, financial, etc.)?
5. "*So what*?" That is, confirm the usefulness of the research. As mentioned, organizations that fund projects, ethics committees will be interested in how these results will be useful.

If you have been able to answer the previous questions and the topic is still current, you must proceed to formulate the research problem, which must be reduced to a single question that can be answered. That single research question is what directs and defines the study [5]. This question is the compass that guides the process, ensuring that we stay focused on the main objective. It is crucial to constantly review it as we go, as it is easy to get sidetracked by new discoveries or emerging data.

2.1.3.1 Finding Gaps in the Knowledge and Research Questions

Before starting any research project, it is essential to carefully review the existing literature to ensure your question is both open and necessary. A good literature review helps avoid redundant efforts, save time and resources, and prevent patient involvement on topics that may have already been resolved or are trivial. By identifying gaps in knowledge, you can target meaningful questions that truly advance the field.

For novice researchers, the discussion sections of recent papers are great places to look for ideas. These often contain phrases like "future research must" or "one question remains," pointing to unexplored areas. Paying attention to these can help ensure your research is relevant, avoid duplication, and maximize its impact.

2.1.3.2 The Research Question

Levi Strauss once stated, "*A scientist is not a person who gives the right answers; they are the one who asks the right questions.*" This highlights the significance of formulating the right questions as the essence of good science, emphasizing its crucial role as the foundation for meaningful research and discovery.

In this regard, there are two important points to consider. The first, already mentioned, is that a well-formulated and regularly reviewed research question is essential for maintaining the focus of the study and for the success of a research project.

Without a clear and well-defined question, a study can lose direction, which could result in scattered and incoherent work. Keeping the question in mind helps align all aspects of the project, from data collection to analysis and interpretation of results. On the other hand, as we saw in the previous section, the answers to the initial research question will generate new questions. This is a natural and expected aspect of the research process. Furthermore, understanding that each answer obtained leads to new questions helps us accept that research is a continuous and dynamic process, always in search of new truth and understanding.

Understanding the attributes of a good question can help identify significant clinical problems that merit research. While experienced researchers find this straightforward, novice researchers often require guidance to navigate the process effectively [6].

Researchers have developed the **PICO** and **FINER** criteria as useful frameworks for developing research questions [6, 7]. Each serves slightly different purposes and can be applied in different contexts within the research process.

The PICO, sometimes with a "T" (i.e., PICOT) to denote the timeframe, is best suited for clinical research questions, particularly those focused on therapeutic interventions, diagnostic tests, or epidemiological studies. PICO stands for:

- **P**: Patient/Population/Problem
- **I**: Intervention
- **C**: Comparison (if applicable)
- **O**: Outcome

On the other hand, the "FINER" criteria are best suited for qualitative research, exploratory studies, or when considering broader research contexts including social science or policy research. The FINER criteria offer some advantages for evaluating research questions. They enable a thorough assessment of the overall significance beyond clinical, emphasize feasibility and highlight the relevance to enhance engagement, and encourage researchers to consider the ethical implications of their research [6]. FINER states that a research question must be:

- **F**: Feasible
- **I**: Interesting
- **N**: Novel
- **E**: Ethical
- **R**: Relevant

Example of PICO in Dentistry:

Clinical Question: How does the use of a fluoride varnish (intervention) compared to no fluoride treatment (comparison) affect the incidence of dental caries (outcome) in children aged 6 to 12 years (population) in a 12-month period?

Breakdown:

- **P** (Population): Children aged 6 to 12 years
- **I** (Intervention): Use of fluoride varnish
- **C** (Comparison): No fluoride treatment

- **O** (Outcome): Incidence of dental caries
- **T** (Time): 12 months

Complete PICOT Question: "In children aged 5 to 12 years, how does the use of fluoride varnish compared to no fluoride treatment in reducing the incidence of dental caries in a 12-month period?"

The Cochrane Library "At-a-Glance PICO Summaries" is a valuable tool for synthesizing and communicating research evidence in a format that enhances understanding and application in clinical practice [8].

Table 2.1 presents examples of questions in oral health research categorized within each Research Focus and Framework.

Once the research question has been defined, it can be answered using quantitative or qualitative methods. In the health science field, quantitative methods that involve numbers, quantities, and statistics are commonly used. However, these methods do not always answer all research questions, which is why qualitative methods are used. The qualitative methodology is different since it does not use statistics but other methods for data analysis and collection. For example, if we want to know the number of people who used a health service or acquired knowledge or practice after an intervention, we need quantitative methods. However, these methods cannot explain why a person used (or did not use) a health service, or had a change in behavior, etc.

When the focus is not so much on discovering causal relationships, but rather on understanding the nature of a phenomenon as experienced by a human being, we

Table 2.1 Examples of questions in oral health research

Research Focus	Framework	Example Question
Prevalence	CoCoPop (Condition, Context, Population)	What is the prevalence of dental caries in primary school children in urban areas of country?
Diagnosis	PIRDS (Population, Index Test, Reference Test, Diagnosis of Interest)	In children with early signs of tooth decay, how accurate is an artificial intelligence model (Index Test) compared to three expert radiologists (Reference Test) in diagnosing dental caries (Diagnosis of Interest)?
Risk Factors	PECO (Population, Exposure, Comparison, Outcomes)	In adolescents, does high sugar consumption compared to low sugar consumption increase the risk of developing dental caries?
Effectiveness	PICO (Population, Intervention, Comparison, Outcome)	In patients with gingivitis, how effective is laser treatment compared to traditional scaling and root planning in reducing gum inflammation?
Economic Analysis	ECLIPSe (Expectations, Client group, Location, Impact, Professionals, Service)	How does the implementation of a school- based fluoride varnish program impact dental care costs for children in rural schools compared to usual care?
Qualitative Science	PICo (Population, Phenomenon of Interest, Context)	How do adult patients perceive the experience of undergoing full-mouth rehabilitation with dental implants in a public healthcare setting?

refer to qualitative methods. The description of these methodologies goes beyond the objectives of this manual; however, these differences are important, due to the design that will be followed, but also due to the way in which quantitative and qualitative studies are published.

2.2 General Aspects of Scientific Writing

There are several documents that, although related and overlapping, are different and more importantly given their specific objectives, the formats differ in general. Each of them plays a crucial role in the cycle of scientific research, from the conception of the idea to the dissemination of results, and it is essential that researchers understand and recognize their differences, formats, audience, and structure, specific purposes and importance of each document in the development of an investigation.

This is important because, although they are all generated from the same research, the style and approach must be adjusted to satisfy the specific objectives and requirements of each type of document.

2.2.1 *The Research Proposal*

One of these documents is the **research proposal**. This is the first step for any study. A good research idea may not be enough, it is necessary to plan the research well and ask yourself if the resources we have will be enough to carry out your project. If they are sufficient, you can continue with writing the study protocol. If, on the other hand, they are not sufficient, a proposal must be made to apply for research grants (See Fig. 2.2).

The research proposal is a written plan that includes the problem to be investigated and its importance, the question/hypothesis to be answered/tested, and the research methodology to be used. It is an initial document that systematically outlines the research question, objectives, justification, and proposed methodology. This document must include all the information necessary for the reader to evaluate

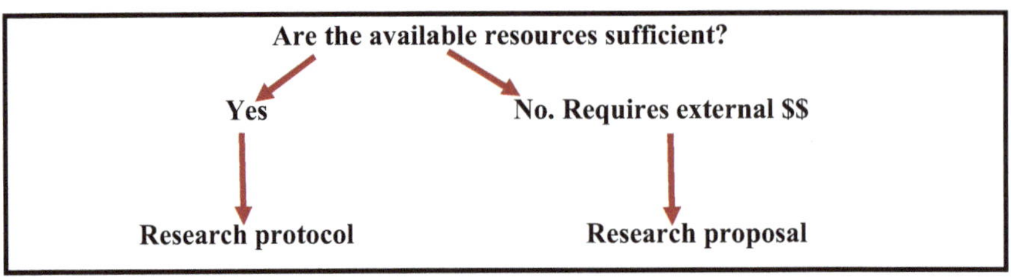

Fig. 2.2 The research proposal-research protocol pathway

the proposed study; it must provide concise and detailed information on each of its components, from the title to the plan for dissemination of results. The research proposal is also used to make presentations and obtain research permits.

A research proposal can have various formats depending on its objectives, such as whether it is intended to be presented to an audience, to an ethics committee, or to request funding. Not all research proposal formats are the same. In each of these cases, the emphasis will be placed on different aspects.

A proposal to request research funds is related but different to the study protocol, as different questions must be answered depending on the funding source. These sources can be:

- Government aid: (e.g., SENECYT, ANID, NH&MRC, etc.)
- Aid from the university system
- Foundations
- Companies (Dental industry)
- Money from the community (e.g., crowdfunding)
- Money from organizations (e.g., NGOs, churches, etc.)

The preparation of a research proposal is an iterative process, which, as opposed to a linear process, includes several cycles. The purpose of the proposal is to ensure that the study is well designed and meets the requirements of the discipline and the institution through which the research will be carried out [9].

Remember that the research proposal will be under rigorous peer scrutiny. The reviewers of the proposals look at elements such as its purpose, the justification and significance of the research (the "*So what?*"), the budget and its justification, whether the project can be carried out in the time and resources proposed, etc.

> A bad idea cannot be transformed into a good proposal. But bad writing can turn a good idea into a poor research proposal [10].

Always keep in mind that, although the research proposal will be read by many experts, they will not necessarily be experts in the area you are researching. Therefore, write in the most general terms possible and do not use uncommonly used technical terms without previously defining them. For example, the Community Periodontal Index (CPI) is widely used in dentistry. However, CPI may mean different things in different professions and contexts. CPI may also refer to Consumer Price Index (Same Term). It is always important to explain the term and its criteria for non-expert readers.

Firstly, always review and familiarize yourself with the research proposal guidelines, standards, instructions, format, and style of the organizations you wish to apply to, as this format varies from one organization to another. Always strictly follow the headings indicated in each case and answer only what they ask of you. Adjust to the requested requirements. For example, word limit, margins, fonts: type and size. If the instructions say, "In no more than 500 words" or "In no more than three pages," do not use more than 500 words or three pages.

In some cases, a limit is placed on the number of references. Always use margins, font sizes, fonts, etc., as indicated.

However, word limits are always important as current writing boxes only allow set words or characters, cutting off words that go beyond the set limit. This is why it is important to follow the indicated format. Consider that, if we exceed the word limit, we are sending the message to those who fund research that we do not pay attention, do not care, do not understand, or do not follow the guidance or instructions to the authors. It is also important to pay attention to each and every element of a research proposal and complete it with the right information in the right place, which is sometimes not easy to achieve.

As formats vary, our intention is not to give a recipe for how to write a proposal. However, despite varying order from institution to institution, research proposals generally have the headings set out in Box 2.1.

Box 2.1 Elements of a Research Protocol and a Research Proposal
Research proposal

- **Title** (concise and effective)
- **Abstract.** A brief summary that summarizes the objectives, methodology, and expectations of the study
- **Aims/objectives/hypothesis**
- **Background** (clear and easy to understand)
  - Justification
  - Literature review
  - Outline of methods
- **Significance**—the "*So what?*"
- **Methodology**
  - Design (aligned to the objectives)
  - Sample

    Sampling
    Sample size (calculation and justification)
  - Data collection.

    Variables to be studied
    Information from the instruments
    Procedures
  - Data analysis.

    Preliminary information on how data will be handled and analyzed
    Alignment with the objectives of study
- **Budget**
  - For key elements and total
  - Justification

(*continued*)

Box 2.1 (continued)

- **Time**
  - Total and by components
- **Expected result:** Although the proposal does not present results, it should detail expectations and how these results will contribute to existing knowledge.
- **Ethical issues.**
  - List and describe the ethical implications of the study and how each of them will be addressed.
  - Data Security & Handling. Details of where records will be kept & how long they will be stored.
- **Strategies for dissemination of results.**
  - Data management plan.
- References

On the other hand, there might be no format. In these situations, follow logical reasoning, that is, keep in mind that a proposal must be presented as an argument that shows logical reasoning for your ideas. Go from the most general to the specific and provide concise and detailed information on each of the components of the project, from the title to the results dissemination plan.

In addition to the scientific validity of a proposal, reviewers look at the following points [11]:

1. The qualifications of the researchers.
2. The experience of the research team:
   a. Previous publications.
   b. Projects in which the research team has participated.
   c. The expertise of the team.
3. The feasibility of the project. Feasibility is not only the ability of the researchers to carry out the research, but also whether they will be able to do it with the money requested and within the established time frame.

2.2.2 *The Research Protocol*

The research protocol, on the other hand, is a more technical working document than the research proposal and is generally not made public [9]. The protocol is a more detailed and specific document than the research proposal, since, in addition to communicating the problem to be investigated, it describes the exact procedures and methods that will be used in the research, to accurately and precisely solve said problem or question, as well as ethical and logistical considerations. This document serves to justify the more technical decisions in relation to the decision making of the project itself; however, its components are the same as those of a research proposal. This document is crucial to ensure that research is conducted in a systematic and replicable manner. The research protocol, like the research proposal, is a document that does not present results, but instead details the plan and procedures to follow.

Writing a research protocol is a slow, long, complicated, and iterative process, typically involving multiple drafts. This process must:

- Include the review of other similar protocols to understand approaches and methodologies.
- Collaborate with experienced colleagues to receive feedback and ensure that the protocol meets scientific standards.
- Ensure that all sections of the protocol are clearly stated and easy to understand.

The proposal must be coherent, well-structured, and justified to demonstrate the feasibility and importance of the proposed study. Furthermore, the protocol must answer three fundamental questions:

1. What is going to be done?
2. How is it going to be done?
3. Why is it going to be done?

Please note that research protocols can also be published. Publication of protocols helps ensure transparency, reproducibility, and dissemination of research methods and findings. Several journals and platforms specifically focus on publishing research protocols. Chapter 5 expands on this.

2.2.3 *The Scientific Publication*

A third type of document is the scientific publication, which is produced at the end of the research since its objective is to communicate and disseminate the results of the study to the scientific community and to the general public.

This is the objective of an investigation: the publication of the results. An experiment or study does not exist until its results have been published [12]. It is only in this way, when the result of the research is subject to evaluation by the scientific community, by peers, that the research exists. As such, the dissemination of results is a fundamental part of all research. Research proposals and protocols are generally not published and, therefore, their readers are a smaller group. In contrast, the dissemination of research results has a broader audience.

Table 2.2 Comparison of a research protocol and the different forms of conference presentation

Abstract	Poster	Oral presentation
250–350 words	(About) 1000 words	12–15 minutes
Title/Author	Title/Author	Title/Author
Introduction	Introduction	Introduction
Objectives	Objectives	(Justification of the problem, bibliography review, theoretical framework, objectives, or initial hypothesis)
Material and Methods	Material and Methods	Material and Methods
Results	Results	Results
Discussion/ Conclusions	Discussion	Discussion
References	Conclusions	Conclusions
	References	References
	Appendices such as: Tables, Figures, Instruments, Surveys, Photos, etc.	Appendices such as: Tables, Figures, Instruments, Surveys, Photos, etc.

Your audience can be as wide as the "world wide web" allows. Among the possible methods for disseminating the results are:

- Conferences—Oral presentation at a conference. This is the presentation of research, findings, or academic works before a specialized audience in a specific field. They usually have a limited duration and are held in the context of conferences, symposiums, or scientific meetings.
- Conferences—Written presentations or posters at a conference. This is the use of visual formats to communicate research findings at conferences and scientific meetings.

Table 2.2 presents a comparison of the different forms of presentation at a conference and their particularities and differences.

- A thesis: the oral presentation or defense of a thesis. They are fundamental components in the process of obtaining a graduate degree, such as a master's degree or doctorate. It involves the oral presentation of the research carried out as part of the thesis before an academic evaluation committee.
- Publications in scientific journals that use more formal formats that communicate the results of the research to the scientific community, following specific structures such as Introduction, Methods, Results, and Discussion (IMRaD).

A manuscript in a scientific journal itself represents a summary of original research that is subject to the publication standards of the journal in which it is presented. In general, a publication has a word limit that is between 3000 and 3500 words, where years of work must be summarized. This is why it can be considered somewhat challenging. New knowledge is communicated and presented in condensed form, providing background information that allows the work to be reproduced. Chapters 6–10 describe in more detail the elements that make up a scientific article.

Three questions to publish in a journal:

1. What is the purpose of the manuscript that I am going to publish. What is my story? Has it been written before?
2. Who is interested?
3. Where will I publish my article?

One possibility is to identify the most cited journal in one's reference list, as it will determine the chances of publication acceptance and the impact of their research. By aligning themselves with the characteristics and approaches that the journal values, and studying its recent trends, researchers can optimize their chances of publication in an academic journal.

Depending on the answer to these three questions, we will be successful in publishing our work.

In addition, there are other documents that may summarize the main findings and conclusions of the research. These are intended for a broader audience in the form of technical reports that provide a detailed analysis of technical aspects of the research. For example:

- Reports
- Publications in weekly or daily newspapers
- Interviews on radio and television
- Online and social media discussions
- Discussions with community members
- Chapters in books
- A book

Writing a scientific publication begins long before the words are put on paper. This initial process is known as prewriting. It is a crucial phase which lays the foundation for a successful publication. This phase is where we prepare for publication, plan our story, identify our target audience, and familiarize ourselves with the submission guidelines and specific formats required by the selected magazine or publication medium. During prewriting, we can also improve grammar and learn techniques to avoid procrastination and make better use of our time.

Table 2.3 presents a comparison of various forms of publications, highlighting their main features, characteristics, and differences.

2.3 Plagiarism

A research paper presents the results of an investigation that is unique and one's own. It is based on one's own thoughts, but also on facts and ideas that have been obtained from different sources.

Table 2.3 Comparison of the different forms of publication

Protocol	Thesis	Manuscript
10,000 words	30,000 words	3000 words
Title	Title	Title
Index	Index	Index
Abstract	Abstract	Abstract
Introduction	Introduction	Introduction
(Justification of the problem, literature review, theoretical framework, objectives or initial hypothesis)	(Justification of the problem, literature review, theoretical framework, objectives or initial hypothesis)	(Justification of the problem, literature review, theoretical framework, objectives or initial hypothesis)
Material and Methods	Material and Methods	Material and Methods
Work plan and Timetable	Results	Results
Budget or necessary resources	Discussion	Discussion/Conclusions
References	Conclusions	References
	References	
	Appendices such as: Tables, Figures, Instruments, Surveys, Photos, etc.	

The use of others' ideas or phrases and pretending that they reflect our own thoughts, either by neglect or intent, is a serious offense called "Plagiarism."

- *"Ideas or phrases"* refers to any materials, written or spoken, ranging from complete sentences and paragraphs to full articles.
- *"Of others"* refers to any source: papers, books, magazines, newspapers, journals, electronic resources, other students, etc. However, this does not only apply to ideas or phrases; indeed, the use of any creative work of others without due acknowledgment of the source is plagiarism [13].
- *"Creative work"* includes published and unpublished written documents, software, designs, music, sounds, images, photographs, ideas, or the ideological frameworks
- Obtained through the work of another person or group. These works can be printed on paper or recorded on electronic media.

Plagiarism is the intentional or unintentional use of the work of others, copying (in full or in part) the work or data of others or presenting substantial extracts from print media, electronic, or other written form, oral, electronic/online or work group, etc., without due recognition [14].

Plagiarism, or rather the duplication of text, is an aspect that is carefully reviewed in manuscripts through various specialized applications. Currently, there are software tools and resources used to detect electronic plagiarism and text duplication. This software compares texts located on the Internet with the text in question, identifying similarities and possible duplications.

Regarding textual quotations, they should be used with caution due to duplication of texts, ensuring that it is related to the topic of each paragraph and citing other sources to support the arguments, and considering the possibility of paraphrasing or rewriting information to avoid duplication. If a certain percentage of duplication is exceeded (for example, 30%), it could indicate originality problems and would be considered plagiarism. To avoid this, you can paraphrase or rewrite the information in a different way, always citing the source.

However, there are cases in which textual citations cannot be avoided, such as when explaining something specific, or using an index, or methodology that cannot be explained in any other way. For example, there are not many different ways to explain the Decay, Missing, and filled (DMF) index. Due to these situations, academic journals use acceptable plagiarism percentage thresholds (for example, 30%) that vary depending on the journal. These thresholds allow for a certain amount of unavoidable duplication, while ensuring that the original content remains intact and that ethical publishing standards are respected. Therefore, it is always important to check for duplication of information, cite the source properly, and check for replication of information using specialized software.

In short, most cases of plagiarism can be avoided by citing the source. Simply acknowledging that the material has been borrowed and providing the reader or audience with the information necessary to find that source is sufficient, in most cases, to prevent plagiarism. To avoid it, referencing methods are used to give recognition to the authors of those ideas, phrases, or thoughts.

References

1. Oxford Learner's Dictionaries. https://www.oxfordlearnersdictionaries.com/ Accessed 12 October 2024.
2. Borbasi S, Langford R, Jackson D. Navigating the maze of nursing research: an interactive learning adventure. Elsevier Australia; 2003.
3. Leedy PD, Ormrod JE. Practical research planning and design. 9th ed. Upper Saddle River, NJ: Pearson Education; 2009.
4. Polgar S, Thomas S. Introduction to research in the health sciences. 6th ed. Churchill Livingstone/Elsevier; 2008.
5. Roberts K, Taylor B. Nursing research processes: An australian perspective. 2nd ed. Nelson; 2001.
6. Thabane L, Thomas T, Ye C, Paul J. Posing the research question: not so simple. Can J Anaesth. 2009;56:71–9. https://doi.org/10.1007/s12630-008-9007-4.
7. Stillwell SB, Fineout-Overholt E, Melnyk BM, Williamson KM. Evidence-based practice, step by step: asking the clinical question: a key step in evidence-based practice. Am J Nurs. 2010;110:58–61. https://doi.org/10.1097/01.NAJ.0000368959.11129.79.
8. Cochrane Library. What is PICO? https://www.cochranelibrary.com/about-pico. Accessed 4 November 2024.
9. Blaikie N. Designing social research: the logic of anticipation. 2nd ed. Polity Press; 2009.
10. Reif-Lehrer L. Grant application Writer's handbook. 3rd ed. Jones & Bartlett Learning; 1995.

11. Naylor C, Williams J, Guyatt G. Structured abstracts of proposals for clinical and epidemiological studies. J Clin Epidemiol. 1991;44:731–7. https://doi.org/10.1016/0895-4356(91)90123-q.
12. Day RA, Gastel B. How to write and publish a scientific paper. 6th ed. Cambridge University Press; 2006.
13. Melbourne University. Academic integrity and plagiarism. http://academichonesty.unimelb.edu.au/2024. Accessed 4 November 2024.
14. University of New England. Plagiarism. https://www.une.edu.au/library/students/referencing-and-plagiarism/plagiarism 2024 Accessed 4 November 2024.

Chapter 3
Administrative Aspects

Ebingen Villavicencio-Caparó and Estefanía Patiño-Ramón

3.1 Introduction

This chapter describes the administrative aspects of bibliographic indexing, emphasizing the evolution of research methodologies in health services. It begins with a historical perspective, highlighting the contributions of Scottish epidemiologist Archie Cochrane, whose work in the 1970s underscored the necessity for evidence-based interventions in healthcare. This led to the development of systematic review techniques and the modernization of bibliographic indexing systems, transitioning from traditional methods like Index Medicus to more sophisticated frameworks established by the Institute for Scientific Information, founded by Eugene Garfield. The chapter discusses the critical role of metadata in enhancing the traceability and management of scientific publications. Metadata, defined as structured data that organizes and facilitates the search for scientific information, is essential for improving the accessibility of research outputs. Key components of metadata include article titles, authorship, abstracts, keywords, publication dates, and Digital Object Identifiers (DOIs). These elements not only aid in the classification and retrieval of articles, but also contribute to the overall integrity and visibility of scientific literature. The chapter concludes by underscoring the importance of robust bibliographic indexing systems in supporting effective health interventions and advancing the field of evidence-based medicine. Through a comprehensive understanding of these

E. Villavicencio-Caparó (✉)
Universidad Católica de Cuenca, Cuenca, Ecuador

Universidad Peruana Cayetano Heredia, Lima, Perú
e-mail: evillavicencioc@ucacue.edu.ec

E. Patiño-Ramón
Universidad Católica de Cuenca, Cuenca, Ecuador
e-mail: erika.patino@est.ucacue.edu.ec

R. Mariño et al. (eds.), *Scientific Writing and Publication Strategies for Oral Health Professionals*, https://doi.org/10.1007/978-3-031-97916-3_3

administrative aspects, researchers and practitioners can better navigate the complexities of scientific communication and enhance the impact of their work in the healthcare domain.

3.2 Introduction to Journal Indexing

Science is the current paradigm of knowledge. In the 1970s, a Scottish epidemiologist, Archie Cochrane, published a book called Effectiveness and Efficacy: Random Reflections on Health Services, in which he stated that health systems always have limited resources so that interventions for patients should be suitable. Their efficacy should be demonstrated using properly designed research [1]. This is how the systematic review technique was born and with it, the need to improve and modernize the bibliographic indexing systems, which up to that time corresponded to Index Medicus and which, thanks to Garfield and the creation of the "Institute for Scientific Information," made it possible to track bibliographic citations, which later led to the creation of the indicator called impact factor [2].

3.3 Understanding Metadata in Scientific Research

There are several mechanisms for the improvement of publication traceability, including the preservation of metadata [3]. These consist of a set of structured data that provides information allowing the organization, search, and management of scientific information [3, 4]. Metadata is a set of structured data that provides information that enables the organization, search, and management of scientific information [3].

Metadata shared by various search engines are:

- Article title: Provides the name of the published article.
- Authors: Lists the article's authors, including their institutional affiliations.
- Abstract: Briefly describes the article's content, including the objectives, methods, results, and primary conclusions.
- Keywords: Specific terms that describe the article's central themes and concepts facilitating its search and classification
- Publication Date: Date that the article was published in the journal.
- DOI (Digital Object Identifier): A unique identifier providing a consistent online link to the article.
- Journal Volume and Number: Information about the specific volume and number of the journal in which the article was published.
- Pages: The range of pages in which the article appears within the journal.
- Bibliographic Reference: Full citation of the article, which may include additional information such as the publisher and ISSN of the journal.

- Categories and Discipline: Classification of the article according to its thematic area or scientific discipline.
- License and Copyright: Information about the license under which the article is published and associated copyright.

Bibliographic reference management software allows metadata to be assigned to a document downloaded from the web.

3.4 e-Tools in Scientific Research

3.4.1 Article Repositories

Article repositories on the web link metadata to the DOI number of each article and they store article files in PDF, HTML, or another format. They are repositories, for example:

- Medline
- SciELO (Scientific Electronic Library Online)
- AJOL (African Journals Online)
- AAS (Asian Academic Society)
- Redalyc (Red de Revistas Científicas de América Latina y el Caribe, España y Portugal)
- DOAJ (Directory of Open Access Journals)
- J-STAGE (Japan Science and Technology Information Aggregator, Electronic)
- ERIC (Education Resources Information Center)

Journals generally use open-access software called OJS, or "Open Journal System," which allows them to act as a repository exclusive to that journal and aids in the management of the metadata of its publications.

3.4.2 Search Engines

Search engines are software tools that enable the search and download of information from all over the web (repositories, journals, websites, and others) and provide links to access the documents stored on each site. They are search engines, for example:

- Google Scholar
- PubMed
- Lilacs
- Scopus
- Web of Science

- APA PscyINFO
- Microsoft Academic
- BASE (Bielefeld Academic Search Engine)
- CORE (COnnecting REpositories)
- Science.gov of the US government
- Semantic Scholar
- SciELO (Scientific Electronic Library Online)
- AJOL (African Journals Online)
- AAS (Asian Academic Society)
- Redalyc (Red de Revistas Científicas de América Latina y el Caribe, España y Portugal)
- DOAJ (Directory of Open-Access Journals)
- J-STAGE (Japan Science and Technology Information Aggregator, Electronic)
- ERIC (Education Resources Information Center)

3.4.3 Keywords

Keywords are used to search for information in both repositories and search engines these are words or phrases that belong to a list of records that make up a thesaurus, which allows for systematic taxonomy and sorting of the keywords that will be used to search for information. Well-known examples are:

- MESH (Medical Subject Heading)
- DECS (Health Descriptors)
- UNESCO Thesaurus
- APA Thesaurus

The criteria used as keywords are combined, as each keyword has its definition, details, and numerical codification.

The different thesauri contain many interoperable terms, but each has a specific terminology. In that sense, using the specific thesaurus recommended by each search engine is ideal.

3.5 Identification Numbers in Scientific Publication

3.5.1 ORCID (Open Researcher and Contributor ID)

ORCID is a unique identifier for researchers and academics. It allows authors to distinguish and link their work precisely. It can incorporate information about the place of work, qualifications, and participation in competitive research funds. It is beneficial for identifying research collaborators worldwide.

It is a number composed of 16 digits, of which the first four are zeros 0000, then eight digits are assigned sequentially. The last four digits can be numbers followed by an X. The URL of the ORCID website https://orcid.org/ is prefixed to this number [5].

ORCID is a valuable tool that provides a unique identity, facilitates visibility and recognition in the academic environment, and contributes to efficiently managing researchers' careers. Furthermore, it is important in academia and science for the following reasons [5]:

- Unique and Accurate Identification: ORCID provides a unique identifier that avoids confusion between researchers with similar or the same names. This code number ensures that publications and scholarly contributions are correctly associated with the corresponding author.
- Academic Output Tracking: The ORCID profile allows researchers to gather all of the publications, peer-review activities, and projects they have participated in one place, which facilitates career tracking and visibility.
- Cross-platform interoperability: ORCID integrates with academic databases, university management systems, and publishing platforms (such as Scopus, CrossRef, or ResearchGate), simplifying the registration and data update processes. By logging into ORCID, researchers can automatically update their scholarly output on various platforms.
- International Recognition and Credibility: ORCID is widely recognized in academia, and many journals and institutions require it for article submission, which increases researchers' visibility and credibility.
- Ease of Application and Funding Processes: By bringing together all academic output in one place, ORCID facilitates the application process for funding or program applications, as it acts as an up-to-date and verifiable portfolio.

3.5.2 ISSN (International Standard Serial Number)

ISSN is a unique identifier for serial publications, such as magazines and newspapers [6]. It facilitates the management and search of these publications. Through the governing body of science, each country's government collaborates with the ISSN identification of the journals published in their country. The first step is to register in the ISSN system by searching on the website for an authorized registration center https://www.issn.org/

The ISSN is important for several key reasons:

- Unique Identification: Each ISSN is unique to a specific journal, avoiding confusion with similarly named publications. This number is crucial for correctly identifying a source in catalogs, research databases, and rankings [6].
- Standardization and Access: Facilitates cataloging in libraries and international databases, such as Scopus or PubMed, ensuring that readers and researchers can quickly locate a specific journal in global databases [6].

- Visibility and Credibility: Increases the credibility of a publication, as ISSN is an internationally recognized standard. Many academic and research institutions require journals to be indexed with an ISSN for inclusion in scientific databases and evaluations [6].
- Ease of Electronic Search and Access: This contributes to the digital organization of publications, allowing search and access systems (such as Google Scholar or university libraries) to quickly identify electronic and physical editions of a journal [6].
- Academic Impact Tracking: The ISSN allows monitoring of a journal's impact and usage in the academic world. Impact indices and publication metrics often require an ISSN to analyze the frequency and influence of publications [6].

3.5.3 ISBN (International Standard Book Number)

ISBN uniquely identifies printed and digital books. It helps in the identification and marketing of books. Until 2007, this number consisted of 10 digits but from that year onward had a 13-digit code (see Fig. 3.1) [7]. The website of the international agency for the ISBN is https://www.isbn-international.org/es

3.5.4 DOI (Digital Object Identifier)

DOI is a unique identifier for digital objects such as journal articles, book chapters, and datasets. It ensures a permanent link to these resources [8].

A DOI is composed of an alphanumeric string that is divided into three main parts (Fig. 3.2):

Fig. 3.1 Barcode of an ISBN [7]. A: the mandatory prefix, currently 978, B: the identification number of the country or linguistic area encoded (between 1 and 5 digits), C: identification of the publisher or imprint registering the book (up to 7 digits), D: publication element, indicating a particular edition and format, E: the rest of the code is mathematically validated

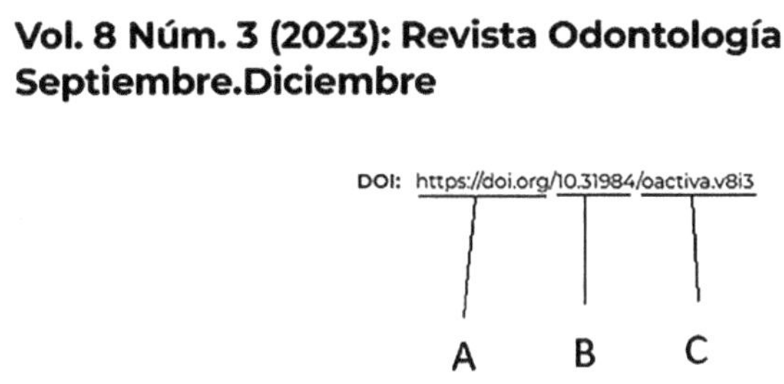

Fig. 3.2 DOI of a journal issue [8]. A: Beginning of the link: "https://doi.org/." All DOIs should begin with this phrase, B: Prefix: This prefix identifies the registering entity (e.g., a publisher or an organization). It usually begins with "10" followed by a series of numbers. In the example, the number 10.31984 belongs to the journal Active Dentistry, C: Suffix: Specifies the particular object and is defined by the registering party. It can contain letters, numbers, hyphens, and other characters. In the example, OACTIVA is the abbreviated name of the journal and V8i3 stands for Volume 8, issue 3

3.5.4.1 Why Is the DOI Number Important?

- Stability and Permanence: Unlike URLs, the DOI remains constant over time. Even if an article changes website or platform, its DOI remains the same, facilitating long-term access.
- Ease of Citation: This facilitates accurate citation of scholarly sources. The DOI is a reliable source for locating the original document without link errors in articles and references [8].
- Interoperability: It is compatible with reference management systems (such as EndNote or Zotero), enabling more manageable and efficient research integration and organization of sources [8].
- Traceability: Facilitates citation tracking, as academic indexing systems use DOIs to track the impact and citations of published works [8].
- Access to Metrics: The DOI contributes to the analysis of citations and impact metrics, which are fundamental in evaluating the quality and scope of research [8].
- Using the DOI in scholarly references ensures reliable accessibility and maintains access to scientific content.

3.5.5 The Author's Signature

Having a unique identification in publications is essential to improve visibility and scientific prestige in the academic world, for both the author and the institution to which the publication belongs.

Why standardize the author's signature? In this image the author appears in PubMed in two distinct formats:

> Villavicencio Caparó E (in Spanish the accent is permitted).
>
> Villavicencio-Caparo E (in English, which does not support the accent).

By not standardizing the signature as an author, our entire scientific production appears to come from diverse sources, when all of it corresponds to a single author. By not standardizing our signature as authors, we are creating diversity in the way we publish, and we may lose some of the works under our authorship [9].

Standardizing the author's signature means choosing a single form in which all your publications should be signed. Search engines support up to 2 different forms of your author signature. Let's look at the example of Google Scholar: https://scholar.google.com/

1. Click on the "Sign in" button in the upper right corner.
2. Sign in with your Google (Gmail) account or create one if you do not already have one.
3. Go to "My profile":
4. Once logged in, click "My Profile" in the upper left corner of the screen.
5. Fill in your personal information:
    - (a) Full Name: Use your professional name, as it will appear in your publications.
    - (b) Affiliation: Specify the institution or university with which you are associated. It is best not to use acronyms.
    - (c) Area of interest: Indicate your areas of research or academic interest.
    - (d) Email for verification: Use your institutional email address (ending in .edu, .org, etc.) to verify your profile.

You will then receive an email from Google Scholar to your institutional email confirming the creation of your account. Finally, the program will automatically recognize and add your publications to your profile. As other authors cite your publications, Google Scholar will indicate year by year how many citations your publications receive. This tool will increase your Google Scholar h-index [10].

Other search engines that allow you to create your user are SCOPUS ID [11] and Web of Science, which can be linked to ORCID.

An important aspect of these profiles is the researcher's photo. A photo should be chosen that conveys professionalism as it is the same one that will be used for the databases mentioned. It should be relatively close and of a more serious nature, and the background should be as plain and clear as possible.

One disadvantage of Google Scholar is that every time we update our profile, it can register as the research of other authors of the same name. Because of this, it is necessary for authors to act ethically and delete any articles that are assigned as theirs and do not belong to them.

For this reason, it is usually better to manually add articles to one's Google Scholar profile rather than doing it automatically.

Now that we have authorship metrics, we are able to observe the historical indicators and citations in general for as long as the author has been publishing and also for the last 5 years.

A profile on Google Scholar amplifies the visibility and impact of academic work, facilitates research career management, and is a tool that supports scientific career development for several reasons:

- Visibility and Accessibility: Google Scholar is one of the most consulted academic platforms in the world, which increases the visibility of publications. Having a profile makes it easier for other researchers to find an author's work in academic search results, improving the reach and impact of their research.
- Impact Metrics: The profile provides statistics, such as the h-index and the i10 index, which help measure publications' influence. These metrics are helpful in impact assessments and can support funding applications or career advancement.
- Citation Tracking: Google Scholar automatically records each publication's citations, allowing the researcher to see how their work contributes to other studies and generates new knowledge.
- Centralization of Publications: The profile consolidates all scientific production in one place, making it easy for others to access and organize academic work. Google Scholar allows you to add articles, correct references, and keep your profile current.
- Professional Recognition: By submitting a profile to Google Scholar, researchers display an academic "business card" on an internationally recognized platform, which can enhance their reputation and professional connections.

  Another fundamental tool for researchers is ResearchGate, which promotes visibility and collaboration, provides relevant metrics, and facilitates access to academic resources, all of which are beneficial for scientific career development; creating a profile on this site offers several advantages for researchers, particularly in terms of visibility, collaboration, and access to academic resources:
- Global Visibility and Networking: ResearchGate connects researchers worldwide, increasing their work's visibility and facilitating networking and interdisciplinary collaborations. Profiles also allow researchers to discover other work related to their field and connect with colleagues.
- Access to Scientific Publications: ResearchGate allows researchers to upload versions of their publications for free sharing, facilitating access to research that may be behind paywalls on other platforms. This is particularly useful in Open Access contexts.
- Metrics and Impact Tracking: The profile provides metrics on paper views, downloads, and citations, allowing researchers to track the reach and influence of their publications. In addition, ResearchGate calculates the Research Interest

Score, an indicator based on interaction with your profile that helps assess the interest generated.
- Constant Updating of the Academic Profile: Researchers can centralize and update all their scientific production in one place, with the option to add preprints, reviews, and data from ongoing projects. This presents a complete and up-to-date picture of their professional trajectory.
- Participation in the Scientific Community: ResearchGate allows you to ask and answer research questions, which fosters knowledge sharing and collaborative learning. Researchers can obtain feedback from other academics and resolve doubts in their areas of interest.

Finally, Publons is a Web of Science (Clarivate Analytics) platform that allows researchers and academics to manage and receive recognition for their peer review and scholarly journal editing activities. It is a tool designed to increase transparency and visibility in the academic review process while recognizing the work of researchers in this area. The main functions and advantages of Publons are:

- Registration of Peer Review Activities: Researchers can register their peer reviews for various journals, allowing them to receive public recognition for this key scientific activity.
- Creation of a Complete Profile: Researchers can aggregate their publications, reviews, and editorial activities into a single profile, providing a complete view of their scientific contribution. This is useful for professional development, as it allows other academics and institutions to see the scope of the researcher's work.
- Metrics and Recognition of Scholarly Contributions: Publons provides metrics and statistics on review activity and publication output, which are increasingly valued by academic institutions as well as promotion and funding committees.
- Collaboration and Networking: By joining Publons, researchers can connect with colleagues, see who has reviewed or edited their articles, and collaborate with other experts in their field.

Publons integrates peer review and editing with publication visibility, which offers a significant advantage in consolidating the prestige and professional recognition of academic researchers.

3.6 Final Remarks

Bibliographic indexing plays a critical role in the health services sector. This chapter provided a comprehensive understanding of bibliographic indexing's administrative aspects, which will enable researchers and practitioners to maximize their work's impact, by improving its accessibility and visibility, ultimately contributing to better health outcomes and informed decision-making in healthcare. A commitment to improving bibliographic practice ensures that knowledge generated in the health sciences field remains accessible and impactful for all those interested in pursuing better health outcomes.

References

1. Cochrane community. Archie Cochrane: the name behind Cochrane https://community.cochrane.org/archie-cochrane-name-behind-cochrane. Accessed 20 July 2024.
2. Garfield E. The history and meaning of the journal impact factor. JAMA. 2006;295:90–3. https://doi.org/10.1001/jama.295.1.90.
3. Pacheco A, Da Silva C, De Freitas M. A metadata model for authenticity in digital archival descriptions. Arch Sci. 2023;23:629–73. https://doi.org/10.1007/s10502-023-09422-w.
4. Paperpile Reference Manager. Paperpile. https://paperpile.com/. Accessed 11 September 2024.
5. ORCID. Available from: https://orcid.org/. Accessed 11 September 2024.
6. International Standard Serial Number. https://www.issn.org/. Accessed 11 September 2024.
7. International Standard Book Number. ¿Qué es un ISBN? 2014. https://www.isbn-international.org/es/content/que-es-un-isbn/10. Accessed 30 July 2024.
8. DOI Foundation. Digital Object Identifier. 2022. https://www.doi.org/. Accessed 11 September 2024.
9. National Center for Biotechnology Information (NCBI). Villavicencio Caparo E - Search Results. PubMed. (1996) 2024. https://pubmed.ncbi.nlm.nih.gov/?term=Villavicencio+Caparo+E. Accessed 11 September.
10. Google Scholar. Google Scholar. 2004. Available from: https://scholar.google.com/. Accessed 12 July 2024.
11. Elsevier. Scopus tutorials - Scopus: Access and use Support Center. 2024. https://service.elsevier.com/app/answers/detail/a_id/14799/supporthub/scopus/#doc. Accessed 11 September 2024.

Chapter 4
Publication Types: Diversifying Scholarly Communication

Sergio E. Uribe

4.1 Introduction

It's common to encounter the phrase "according to a study …" in news reports, accompanied by some data reported in a manuscript. However, various articles or studies can be published in a scientific journal, with the strength of evidence ranging from simple opinions to large-scale scientific studies involving thousands of patients. These studies can be crucial for identifying the effects of medical interventions. Therefore, "I read it in a scientific journal" often requires clarification.

In addition, "according to a study" is a phrase that is as overused as it is inaccurate: not everything that journals publish is a study, nor have all their articles been peer-reviewed. Like in traditional media, there are different genres, and scientific publications range from letters and editorials to proper scientific reports. In this chapter, you will discover the most common types of publications found in scientific journals and the usual structure or content of a typical scientific article. But first, we will discuss the scientific cycle to give a general perspective.

4.2 The Cycle of Science

Figure 4.1 shows "The Science Cycle," highlighting the stages of Research Protocol, Data, and Communication as key steps in the research process.

S. E. Uribe (✉)
Department of Conservative Dentistry and Oral Health, Riga Stradins University, Riga, Latvia

Department of Conservative Dentistry, Periodontology and Digital Dentistry, LMU University Hospital, LMU Munich, Germany
e-mail: sergio.uribe@rsu.lv

R. Mariño et al. (eds.), *Scientific Writing and Publication Strategies for Oral Health Professionals*, https://doi.org/10.1007/978-3-031-97916-3_4

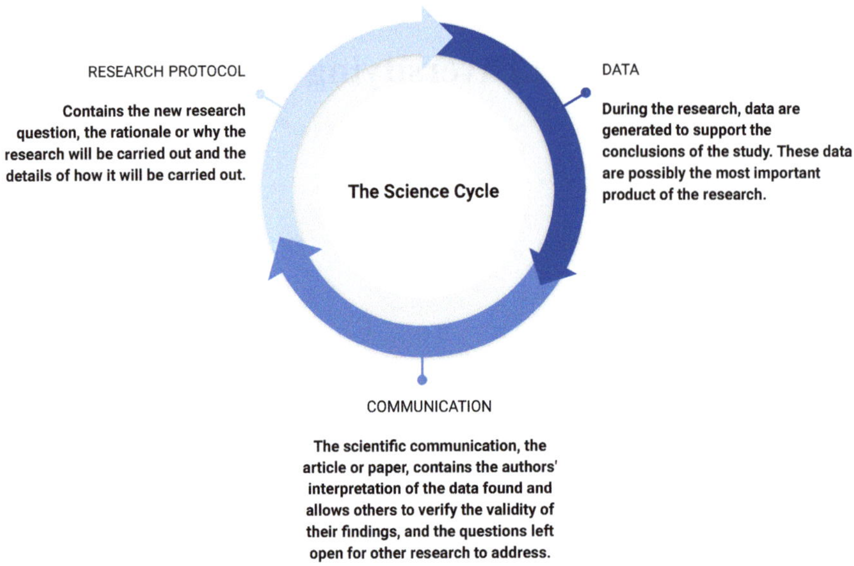

Fig. 4.1 The cycle of science

Table 4.1 Key benefits of publishing research protocols

Benefit	Description
Establishing Credibility and Expertise	Publishing protocols allow researchers to showcase expertise in a specific methodology, enhancing their reputation and visibility. They also demonstrate transparency and rigor, which are valued qualities often leading to more citations and collaboration opportunities.
Protecting Intellectual Property	Documenting the study design in a protocol publication helps establish intellectual ownership, ensuring researchers are credited for their contributions before the study is completed.
Promoting Accountability and Reducing Bias	Publicly available protocols promote accountability by adhering to a predefined approach, reducing selective reporting. This is crucial in clinical and experimental research, ensuring that reported findings reflect the original study design.

Publishing the protocol also benefits researchers; some of these advantages are summarized in Table 4.1.

4.2.1 The Research Protocol

The science cycle illustrates the steps from the conception of an idea to its scientific communication, beginning with a research question. In this stage, researchers decide to pursue the answer to a scientific query. Dental research involves multiple individuals, equipment, and resources. Detailed planning is essential, including securing funding, given the complexity and investment involved. This entire plan is formally documented in a **research protocol**—a comprehensive document detailing the study's purpose, objectives, methodology, and planned analyses.

4.2.1.1 Publishing the Research Protocol

Publishing the Research Protocol is an increasingly recognized and valued step in scientific research. By publicly sharing the protocol, researchers provide a transparent study roadmap, enabling the scientific community to understand, replicate, and build on the methodology. This publication often marks the first formal record associated with a specific research project, establishing the study's credibility.

Publishing research protocols has far-reaching implications for the advancement of science:

1. **Establishing Transparency and Rigor**: A published protocol enhances transparency by clarifying the study's objectives, planned methods, and analyses ahead of time. This reduces the risk of introducing bias through unplanned changes during or after data collection, thereby enhancing the scientific rigor of the study. This commitment to a predefined approach strengthens not only the study's validity, but also the credibility of the researchers.
2. **Prevention of Redundant Research Efforts**: By making protocols publicly available, researchers help prevent unnecessary duplication of efforts. Others can easily find and assess the study plan, potentially avoiding repeated work in fields with limited resources. Furthermore, transparency fosters opportunities for collaboration among researchers with aligned goals, facilitating a more efficient path toward discovery.
3. **Early Peer Input and Methodological Refinement**: When researchers publish protocols before beginning data collection, they open the door to early feedback from the scientific community. This feedback can refine the study's methodology and improve its design, enhancing the findings' quality and impact. This openness to critique also aligns with broader movements toward open science, where early peer input is encouraged.

4.2.1.2 Components of a Research Protocol

The research protocol is a comprehensive document that provides all essential details about a research study, serving as a roadmap from concept to completion. A well-constructed protocol assures readers, collaborators, and reviewers that:

1. The study is carefully designed with clear objectives, significance, and contributions.
2. The research team possesses the necessary background and expertise.
3. There are adequate resources and support systems to carry out the study.
4. Each project stage, including timelines and funding use, has been thoughtfully planned and outlined.

The protocol document ensures transparency, accountability, and reproducibility by clearly presenting the study's objective, design, methodology, and administrative aspects. The protocol also conveys to stakeholders that, with appropriate support, the research will make a meaningful contribution to its field. The essential components of a research protocol are listed in Table 4.2.

Following the components outlined in Table 4.2, it is crucial to follow **reporting guidelines** like CONSORT for clinical trials, STROBE for observational studies, and PRISMA for systematic reviews. Adhering to these standards ensures clarity, completeness, and transparency, enhancing the quality and reproducibility of the research. Additional resources are available at the EQUATOR Network [2, 3].

Consulting a statistician during the protocol writing phase is essential to ensure rigorous study design, accurate sample size calculation, and a sound data analysis plan, strengthening the study's validity from the outset. As R.A. Fisher, widely regarded as one of the founders of modern statistics, aptly noted, "*To consult the statistician after an experiment is finished is often merely to ask him to conduct a postmortem examination. He can perhaps say what the experiment died of.*" [4].

Where to Publish Research Protocols, research protocols can be published in specialized repositories and journals to enhance transparency and allow for early peer feedback. Common platforms for protocol publication include **Open Science Foundation (OSF)**, **PROSPERO** (for systematic reviews), and **Protocols.io**, both of which support open access and long-term visibility. Additionally, journals such as *BMC Oral Health* and *BMJ Open* accept protocol articles, providing a peer-reviewed format that ensures protocols are accessible and citable. Publishing protocols on these platforms strengthens methodological transparency and helps establish the research's credibility from the outset.

4.2.2 The Research Data

Research data is perhaps a study's most valuable output, providing the foundational evidence to answer the research question. While the manuscript offers one interpretation or analysis, the underlying data is a versatile resource that supports various analyses and interpretations. This flexibility in data use enables other researchers to approach the data from new perspectives, potentially uncovering additional insights or validating original findings.

Moreover, sharing research data ensures that study results can be independently verified, strengthening the applicability and reliability of findings in clinical and scientific practice. When independent researchers have access to well-documented, high-quality data, they can critically assess the methods and conclusions of the original study, perform secondary analyses, or incorporate the data into meta-analyses, advancing scientific knowledge and improving evidence-based applications.

Table 4.2 Essential components of a research protocol

Component	Description
Administrative Data	The protocol title, short title, date, amendment dates, author affiliations, ORCID ids, corresponding author's contact details and funding sources.
Abstract	Provides a concise overview, including background/context, primary and key secondary objectives, study design, setting, participants, data sources, and main outcome measures.
Background	Summarizes the clinical importance of the condition being studied and the significance of the research question, typically in 1–3 sentences.
Objective, Significance, and Hypotheses	Explains the study's main objective, its relevance to the field or society and what the research seeks to demonstrate. Includes any key hypotheses guiding the study.
Study Design	Describes the study's basic design (e.g., retrospective/prospective, cohort, case–control) and setting (e.g., location, inpatient/outpatient, number of sites), ensuring adherence to specific guidelines such as CONSORT for clinical trials or STROBE for observational research [1].
Population and Sample	Defines the target population, sample size assumption based on the hypothesis, eligibility criteria, and participant description.
Interventions/ Exposures	Details any interventions or exposures applied to study groups, if applicable, with guidance from relevant reporting standards such as TIDieR or SPIRIT for clinical trials.
Outcome Measures	Specifies primary and secondary outcome measures and how they will be assessed, with consideration for guidelines such as STARD for diagnostic studies.
Data Collection and Sources	Outlines data collection methods, sources and timing, including data type (e.g., experimental, observational), and collection process, emphasizing compliance with reporting guidelines to ensure transparency and reproducibility.
Data Analysis Plan	Describes statistical methods and approaches for analyzing primary and secondary outcomes, ensuring clear rationale and adherence to appropriate standards.
Data Management Plan	Details data types, formats, metadata, storage, availability, and contact information for queries.
Ethical and Legal Considerations	Summarizes ethical approvals, participant protections and anticipated legal or access restrictions.
Limitations	Identifies potential limitations and anticipated impacts on study findings.
Use of Funds	Outlines how funding will be allocated, specifies anticipated expenses, and demonstrates a well-considered budget.
Researcher Qualifications	Highlights relevant experience, skills, or prior work that positions the researcher to conduct the study successfully.
Dissemination	Details expected venues for sharing findings, including planned publications, conference presentations, or data repositories, to maximize the research's impact and accessibility.

4.3 Types of Data Collection

Two primary distinctions in data collection are **prospective vs. retrospective** and **qualitative vs. quantitative data**, both essential to consider in designing a robust study.

4.3.1 Prospective vs. Retrospective Data

Prospective data collection involves gathering new data based on a predefined study plan. This approach allows for greater control over data quality, as researchers can design and standardize data collection methods to directly align with the study objectives. Prospective studies are particularly valuable when investigating new phenomena, applying precise, controlled methods to observe long-term outcomes or assess causation or evaluate predictions. However, they tend to be more resource-intensive, requiring significant time and financial commitment.

In contrast, **retrospective data** collection relies on existing data from hospital records, clinics, or government databases. Since the data has already been collected, retrospective studies are often faster and more cost-effective. This approach is useful for exploring questions using historical data, identifying trends, evaluating diagnostic devices or conducting large-scale analyses without requiring new data collection. However, retrospective studies can present challenges in data quality control, as the data may lack specific details or standardization needed for the study, and researchers must work within the limitations of the available records.

4.3.2 Qualitative vs. Quantitative Data

Data can also be classified as **qualitative** or **quantitative**, each playing distinct roles in research. **Qualitative data**, such as interview transcripts, case notes, or observational records, captures in-depth, descriptive information and is essential for understanding complex phenomena, behaviors, or motivations. Qualitative data requires careful handling, coding, and thematic analysis to interpret non-numerical insights, making it invaluable in fields like social sciences and behavioral research.

Quantitative data, on the other hand, consists of numerical measurements, statistical records, or other quantifiable information. This data type allows for statistical analysis, pattern identification, and hypothesis testing and is widely applicable in clinical and biomedical research. Quantitative data is often used to establish correlations, predict outcomes, or provide statistical validation of hypotheses.

4.4 Data Management and Planning

In modern research, data is not only a supporting element but a primary research output that should be **as open as possible and as closed as necessary**. This approach aligns with the principles of open science, ensuring that data is accessible to the scientific community while respecting privacy and ethics considerations. Effective data management is essential to prepare data for publication, enabling others to validate findings, conduct secondary analyses, and build on existing knowledge.

To meet these standards, researchers should aim to make data **FAIR**—Findable, Accessible, Interoperable, and Reusable:

1. **Findable**: Data should be easily located with sufficient metadata, often through repositories and indexing.
2. **Accessible**: Data should be openly accessible, with appropriate permissions and controls where necessary.
3. **Interoperable**: Data should be compatible with various systems, tools, and datasets, enabling broad use.
4. **Reusable**: Data should be well-documented and licensed for reuse, ensuring that future researchers can apply it effectively.

A comprehensive **Data Management Plan (DMP)** facilitates these FAIR principles by outlining how data will be organized, stored, and shared throughout the research lifecycle. In Table 4.3, you will find the minimal elements of a DMP.

When combined with other key outputs—such as the research protocol, raw data, and final study report—this approach strengthens open science, providing transparency and accessibility across all stages of research.

Table 4.3 Basic elements of a data management plan

Item	What to include
Data Collection	Types of data
Data Storage	Where and how data will be stored securely
Data Organization	How data will be organized and labeled
Data Access	Who will have access and levels of access permissions
Data Sharing	If, how, and when will data be shared? If not, why will it not be shared
Data Preservation	How data will be preserved for future use or reference. Check Sect. 4.4.1 for where to publish the data.
Ethical Considerations	Compliance with ethical standards regarding data management.

4.4.1 Where to Publish the Data

Researchers are encouraged to publish their data in reputable repositories that ensure long-term accessibility, visibility, and compliance with FAIR standards. Common options include:

1. **General-purpose repositories**: Platforms like **Zenodo**, **Dryad**, **Open Science Framework (OSF)**, and **Figshare** are widely used across disciplines. They allow data to be openly shared with unique DOIs for citation.
2. **Discipline-specific repositories**: For fields like biomedical research, repositories such as **BioStudies** and **GenBank** may be more suitable, as they offer tailored data management features and indexing relevant to specific research areas.
3. **Institutional repositories**: Many universities and research institutions host repositories that provide centralized, long-term storage options and may include tailored support for researchers.

4.5 The Research Article

Finally, researchers communicate the results of their research and their interpretation of the data in a scientific article or paper. This document contains the details of the rationale behind the research, the description of the methods used to collect the data, the summary of the data, and the interpretation of the results. It should allow other researchers to verify the results and clinicians to assess the validity and applicability of the research.

The scientific article can initially be published as a preprint on a preprint server if the results are urgently needed, as was the case with many research papers during the COVID-19 pandemic. Once researchers have conducted their studies and analyzed the data, they prepare a scientific article to communicate their findings. This document serves as a comprehensive research record, enabling others to verify the results and assess their validity and applicability. To ensure the quality and credibility of published research, scientific articles often undergo peer review before being published in a journal.

4.6 Types of Articles You Can Find in a Scientific Journal

A scientific journal can have different articles, but only some are considered scientific. The main characteristic of a scientific article is that it contains all the necessary information to replicate or validate the findings. For this reason, they follow a common structure known as IMRD, which includes an introduction, methods, results, and discussion.

4.6.1 Commonly Accepted Articles in Dental Journals

Table 4.4 lists accepted papers from various dental journals.

All of these journals accept at least three types of papers:

4.6.1.1 Original Research/Research Articles

Original Research or Research Articles present new findings and insights from scientific investigations. These peer-reviewed articles typically include an introduction, methods, results, discussion, and conclusion sections. They aim to contribute new knowledge to the field by describing original experiments, analyses, or studies conducted by the authors. Examples of such articles are found in:

- *Journal of Dental Research*: Maximum 3200 words, five figures/tables, 40 references and a 300-word abstract.
- *Journal of Oral Rehabilitation*: Maximum 2000 words, six figures/tables, 50 references and a 250-word structured abstract.
- *International Journal of Paediatric Dentistry*: Maximum 3500 words (or 5000 for qualitative research), 30 references and divided into sections with detailed methods and results.

4.6.1.2 Reviews/Review Articles

Reviews or Review Articles provide a comprehensive and critical evaluation of existing literature on a specific topic. They are also peer-reviewed, like original research. They aim to summarize and synthesize the current state of knowledge,

Table 4.4 Commonly accepted articles in dental journals

Type of article	Research articles	Letters to the editor	Reviews	Short communications	Other
BMC Oral Health	X		X	Database article, Software article, Case report, Study protocol	
Journal of Dental Research	X	X	X		Debate, Perspective
Journal of Dentistry	X		X	X	Essays (Discovery!)
Dental Traumatology Journal	X	X	X	X	Mini reviews
Journal of Oral Rehabilitation	X	X	X		
Clinical Oral Investigations	X	X	X	X	
Caries Research	X	X	X		Methods article
International Journal of Pediatric Dentistry	X	X	X	X	

highlight key findings, and identify gaps or controversies in the literature. Review articles help researchers stay up to date with recent developments and provide a foundation for future research in the field. Common examples include:

- *Journal of Dental Research*: Critical Reviews in Oral Biology & Medicine section has a maximum of 4000 words, six figures/tables, 60 references and a 300-word abstract. Invitation only.
- *Journal of Oral Rehabilitation:* Structured summary of publication selection with a maximum of 7500 words, six figures/tables and 50 references.
- *International Journal of Pediatric Dentistry:* Invited by the Editor.

4.6.1.3 Letters to the Editor

Letters to the Editor are short communications addressed to the editor of a journal. Letters are not peer-reviewed. They usually raise comments, questions, or concerns about a previously published article or express opinions on a topic of interest. They provide a platform for readers to engage in scientific discourse, share alternative perspectives, or suggest improvements related to published research. Letters to the Editor are typically concise and focused on a single issue or topic. These include:

- *Journal of Dental Research:* Maximum 250 words, no figures/tables. Position on scientific or editorial content.
- *Journal of Oral Rehabilitation:* Comments or questions on published articles with a maximum of 1500 words, 1 figure/table and five references.
- *International Journal of Pediatric Dentistry:* Comments on published articles or new issues with a maximum of 1500 words and ten references.

4.6.2 Other Types of Articles Available in Dental Journals

In addition to the common types of articles such as Original Research, Reviews and Letters to the Editor, some journals also publish other specific articles. Here is a brief description of some of these specific article types and the journals that publish them:

1. **Debate**: Debate articles present opposing viewpoints on controversial or complex topics in a specific field. They provide a platform for experts to discuss and argue different perspectives, enabling readers to understand the subject matter better. The Clinical Oral Investigations journal accepts this kind of article.
2. **Perspective:** Perspective articles offer a personal viewpoint or opinion on a current or relevant topic in the field. They allow authors to share their unique insights, experiences, or ideas, often based on their expertise or research, to stimulate further discussion and development. Clinical Oral Investigations includes these articles under the "Perspective" section, while the Journal of Oral Rehabilitation also features such articles in its publication.

3. **Discovery:** Discovery! Articles are specific to the Journal of Dental Research, focusing on seminal events or advances in dental research. These articles highlight significant breakthroughs, innovations, or milestones that have shaped the field and contributed to its progress. The Journal of Dental Research publishes these articles to showcase the important moments and developments that advance the science of dentistry.
4. **Short Communication or Brief Report:** Short Communications or Brief Reports are concise articles that present new research findings or preliminary results. They are typically shorter than full-length research articles and aim to rapidly disseminate important information, preliminary data, or novel observations that warrant immediate attention. For instance, Clinical Oral Investigations includes these under the "Brief Report" section, while the International Journal of Pediatric Dentistry features them as "Short Communications."
5. **Case Reports:** These describe unique, interesting, or rare clinical cases, often highlighting unusual symptoms, diagnostic challenges, or innovative treatment approaches. They provide valuable insights into real-world clinical situations and contribute to understanding a specific condition or disease. The Journal of Oral Rehabilitation includes Case Reports in its publication, while the International Journal of Pediatric Dentistry features them under the "Brief Clinical Reports/Case Reports" section.

These specific article types cater to the diverse needs of researchers, clinicians, and readers, offering various perspectives and formats to share and disseminate knowledge in the field. It is essential to consult the author guidelines of each journal for detailed information and requirements regarding these specific article types.

4.6.3 Other Types of Scientific Publications

In addition to traditional journal articles, the scientific community engages in various other types of publications to share research findings, data, and methods. These alternative forms of dissemination, **usually not peer-reviewed**, contribute to Open Science, collaboration, and transparency, allowing researchers to access and build upon diverse resources. Here is an overview of some of these other types of publications:

4.6.3.1 Preprint

Before publication, studies may be shared by authors in repositories such as medRxiv, bioRxiv, ResearchSquare, and arXiv. These preliminary papers are known as preprints. They have not passed peer review and can be uploaded with few controls. Some journals and publishers, such as **BMC Oral Health** from Springer, offer authors the option to publish their submitted papers as preprints on platforms like

ResearchSquare. This feature enables the research to be publicly available and citable during the peer-review process, allowing other researchers to reference the work before it's officially published. This practice not only enhances the visibility of new research but also accelerates scientific communication by making findings accessible to the community without delay.

4.6.3.2 Thesis

Original research work carried out by a doctoral student to obtain a professional or academic degree. The thesis must be defended before a panel of examiners. Sometimes, these theses can be the seed that gives rise to one or more articles published in journals after passing peer review.

4.6.3.3 Communication at a Conference

This is a condensed version of a scientific article presented as a presentation or poster to researchers' peers at a conference. It may refer to an already published, peer-reviewed study or advanced preliminary data that is still being worked on.

4.6.3.4 Datasets

Datasets are collections of data, usually organized and structured, that researchers share to facilitate collaboration, transparency, and reproducibility. They can be shared through dedicated repositories, such as Dryad, Figshare, or Zenodo, and may include raw data, processed data, or both.

4.6.3.5 Protocols

Protocols are detailed plans or methods for conducting research, experiments, or clinical trials. They outline the objectives, rationale, design, and procedures of a study, as well as any ethical considerations. Sharing protocols can help promote transparency, reproducibility, and collaboration in research. They can be published in dedicated journals like Nature Protocols and Trials, in specific repositories such as ISRCTN Registry [5] or shared through platforms like Open Science Foundation Registries (OSF) or protocols.io. In addition, some dental journals like BMC Oral Health accept protocols.

These additional publications contribute to the scientific community by providing various formats for sharing research findings, data, and methods and promoting open science, collaboration, and transparency.

4.7 New Ways Scientists Communicate Their Findings

In the digital age, scientists increasingly use new communication channels to share their research and engage with a broader audience. In addition to traditional journal publications, researchers now use blogs, social media, and personal websites to disseminate their work and foster open dialogue.

Blogs allow scientists to present their research in a more accessible and engaging format, often providing context and insights that may not be included in formal publications.

Social media platforms like X (formerly known as-Twitter), LinkedIn, and ResearchGate enable researchers to network, collaborate, and share their findings with a global audience, facilitating rapid knowledge exchange and real-time discussion. **Personal websites** serve as a central hub for scientists to showcase their research, publications and professional achievements. These websites often include easy-to-understand summaries of complex research, making findings more accessible to the general public, policymakers and potential collaborators.

4.8 The Common Objective of Scientific Communication

All forms of scientific communication share a common goal: to enable replication and validation of findings, ensuring the reliability and advancement of research. Transparent communication promotes innovation, accelerates discovery, and promotes collaboration. In the digital age, open access and data sharing increases visibility impact, and collective problem-solving in adhering to this principle, researchers contribute to a transparent and collaborative scientific community that drives progress for the benefit of society.

4.9 Conclusion

Scientific communication encompasses all research outputs that enable the dissemination of research results and ensure their reproducibility and transparency. Traditionally, the research manuscript has been considered the primary research product, but the value of both the research protocol and the research data is now recognized. The use of preprints, non-peer-reviewed documents that allow rapid dissemination of research results, has also become popular in health emergencies such as pandemics. Overall, we now have a variety of ways to disseminate research results and together these different publications can increase the impact of research and ensure that society benefits from the results of science.

References

1. Simera I, Moher D, Hoey J, Schulz KF, Altman DG. A catalogue of reporting guidelines for health research. Eur J Clin Invest. 2010;40:35–53. https://doi.org/10.1111/j.1365-2362.2009.02234.x.
2. Richards D. The EQUATOR network and website. Evid Based Dent. 2007;8:117. https://doi.org/10.1038/sj.ebd.6400533.
3. Moher D, Collins G, Hoffmann T, Glasziou P, Ravaud P, Bian ZX. Reporting on data sharing: executive position of the EQUATOR Network. BMJ. 2024;386:e079694. https://doi.org/10.1136/bmj-2024-079694.
4. Dempfle LRA. Fisher and the development of statistics. J Anim Breed Genet. 2018;135:333–4. https://doi.org/10.1111/jbg.12354.
5. International Standard Randomised Controlled Trial Number (ISRCTN). ISRCTN Registry https://www.isrctn.com/. Accessed 16 November 2024.

Chapter 5
Enhancing Research Transparency: Open Protocols, Access, and FAIR Data

Sergio E. Uribe and Rodrigo Mariño

"Science is like a parachute: it only works when it's open"
—Attributed to many authors

5.1 Introduction

Wilhelm Conrad Roentgen's discovery of X-rays in 1895 marked a advancement in scientific research and medical diagnostics [1]. In his laboratory, Roentgen noticed unexpected images on a photographic plate during experiments with cathode rays, leading him to uncover the mysterious X-rays. Recognizing the significance of his findings, Roentgen documented his experimental setup and methods and shared these details with the scientific community. As a result, researchers and individuals worldwide reproduced his discovery with basic components. A few months later, Otto Walkhoff used this new knowledge to take the first dental radiograph [2]. This

S. E. Uribe (✉)
Department of Conservative Dentistry and Oral Health, Riga Stradins University, Riga, Latvia

Department of Conservative Dentistry, Periodontology and Digital Dentistry, LMU University Hospital, LMU Munich, Germany
e-mail: sergio.uribe@rsu.lv

R. Mariño
Melbourne Dental School, The University of Melbourne, Melbourne, Australia

Center for Research in Epidemiology, Economics and Oral Public Health (CIEESPO), University de la Frontera, Temuco, Chile

Department of Conservative Dentistry and Oral Health, Riga Stradins University, Riga, Latvia

Monash Health Dental Services, Melbourne, Australia
e-mail: r.marino@unimelb.edu.au

R. Mariño et al. (eds.), *Scientific Writing and Publication Strategies for Oral Health Professionals*, https://doi.org/10.1007/978-3-031-97916-3_5

moment in science exemplifies the impact of research and how shared knowledge and data can accelerate innovation and practical applications across borders.

This example is a story of scientific discovery by fortunate coincidence (i.e., serendipitous). There are many such examples in science. However, it also illustrates how the scientific community and society at large can benefit from advancements from research, when they are rapidly disseminated, emphasizing the role of publication of new discoveries throughout the research process. This chapter outlines the advantages of utilizing open protocols for writing research articles, promoting transparency, and enabling other researchers to replicate studies. Additionally, the chapter advocates for the importance of publishing open-access materials, facilitating broader access to research findings, and enabling collaboration among the scientific community. Furthermore, it advocates for the critical role of data repositories that adhere to FAIR principles, ensuring that research data is easily discoverable and usable by others [3].

5.2 The Science Going Backward: From Open to Closed

Science has become competitive among countries, institutions, and researchers. Several factors may have created this culture of secrecy over collaboration, diminishing the cooperative essence once inherent to scientific discovery. Among the reasons for this shift were:

1. **Incentive structures:** Researchers often face significant pressure to publish in high-impact journals, which traditionally operate on subscription models. This competitive environment discourages sharing data and findings before publication, as researchers may fear losing a competitive edge or funding opportunities. The focus on journal publications as a primary measure of success leads to a reluctance to share preliminary results or underlying data, which are crucial for open science practices.
2. **The incentive is placed on the paper rather than the scientific process**: Government bodies provide funding to universities for research activities, which can include paying for the publication of academic papers. As a consequence, university administrations prioritize research outcomes over the scientific process, favoring final publications over the iterative nature of the inquiry and true knowledge building. This emphasis on results can dissuade researchers from sharing methodologies, negative findings, or incremental data, hindering collaborative and transparent science. As a result, the pressure to generate notable publications can encourage practices that favor individual or institutional gain over collective knowledge advancement.
3. **Financial barriers:** Many academic journals charge high subscription fees, limiting access to research for individuals and institutions without sufficient funding. Universities spend millions on journal subscriptions. This results in publicly funded research being accessible only to individuals with access to academic libraries, thus limiting availability to the general public and undermining the fundamental principle of open science.

4. **Cultural resistance:** Some researchers may hesitate to adopt open science practices because of concerns about potential misuse of their data, loss of control over their findings, or the quality of their research being compromised through interpretation by non-experts. These hesitations may impede their willingness to openly share data and collaborate across disciplines.
5. **Lack of infrastructure:** The existing infrastructure for research dissemination does not often support open science. Many researchers lack the necessary tools and platforms to share their work openly. In addition, there is often insufficient institutional support for open science initiatives, including training and resources for researchers to adopt open practices.
6. **Legal and policy constraints:** Intellectual property laws and restrictive publishing agreements can limit researchers' ability to share their work openly. In some cases, legal agreements or ethical considerations may restrict data sharing, particularly in fields involving sensitive information.

However, these pressures have also prompted a movement toward open science. Recent trends in scientific publication business models, along with advancements in technology, have facilitated the transition from the traditional subscription model to more transparent, accessible, equitable scientific publication practices. This shift toward open-access publishing demostrates the necessity to reevaluate our publication practices. It is now possible for research to be freely available for the consumer, although we are currently in a transition phase, yet the two different publication business models still overlap. Factors playing a significant role in facilitating this change are:

(a) **Publication bias**: Commercially funded research may impose the condition of publishing only those results that support their products' efficacy, omitting potentially negative data [4]. This bias distorts scientific truth and can lead to misinformed public health and clinical decisions [4].

(b) **Challenges in scientific communication during health emergencies:** During the COVID-19 pandemic, the urgency to share virus-related discoveries rapidly increased preprint publications, which are not peer-reviewed. While this accelerated information dissemination, it also generated confusion and the spread of unverified data, emphasizing the need to balance speed with rigor during emergencies.

(c) **Recognition that publicly funded data belongs to the public**: There is a growing consensus that results and data from publicly funded research should be accessible to all, not exclusive to those who generate it. This is now a requirement for organizations such as the National Institutes of Health (NIH), European Research Council (ERC), UK Research and Innovation (UKRI), World Health Organization, Science Foundation Ireland and Australia's National Health and Medical Research Council, among others [5]. This approach supports the vision that scientific knowledge should be a common good, free from restricted access that could hinder its dissemination and application for general benefit. However, while there has been progress toward making such information available, we currently find ourselves in a transitional phase before these policies are widely implemented. The term "freely available" is somewhat subjective, as the accessibility of this research is facilitated through funding that supports organizations responsible for disseminating the information to the public.

(d) **Increase in scientific fraud due to misaligned incentives**: The rise in scientific fraud cases and publication retractions emphasize the need for open access to research data for verification purposes. Data availability enables other researchers to replicate and validate studies, essential for maintaining scientific integrity. For instance, replicating studies in psychology and biomedicine has revealed result manipulation or questionable statistical methods, indicating the need for a culture of greater transparency and accountability [6].

In response, major research funding agencies worldwide have begun changing their policies to embrace the principles of open science [5]. These changes aim to recapture the original spirit of scientific inquiry—open, collaborative, and universally beneficial.

5.3 Pros and Cons for Moving to Open Science

Remaining within a closed science model rather than transitioning to an Open Science one may have some detrimental effects on the scientific and academic community and society at large. Here are some of the primary concerns:

1. **Restricted knowledge access:** Closed science limits access to research findings, hindering innovation and informed decision-making in various fields.
2. **Reduced collaboration leading to duplication of research efforts**: Closed science reduces opportunities for collaboration, leading to duplication of research efforts, and missing opportunities for interdisciplinary research opportunities and innovation.
3. **Reproducibility challenges:** Closed science contributes to reproducibility issues due to lack of transparency, making it difficult to validate findings and ensure research reliability.
4. **Inequitable resource distribution:** Closed science does not contribute to equality in access to research and resources, instead widening the gap between well-funded institutions and those with limited resources.
5. **Slows down scientific progress:** Closed science slows scientific advancements by creating knowledge and resource-sharing barriers, particularly in fast-evolving fields like medicine and technology.

On the other hand, article-processing charges (APCs) for authors publishing in open-access journals have become an integral part of the scientific publishing known as open access. In 2025, the editorial boards of two journals resigned in protest for the high APCs, arguing that they exacerbate global inequities as eligibility for fee waivers was often unclear [7].

Arguments in favor of the traditional model by subscription include that it ensures quality control through peer review, which can be compromised in open-access models lacking rigorous standards. The costs associated with subscriptions would be justified by the quality and credibility of the research published in these journals.

Additionally, access to information and data is influenced not only by journal subscription models but also by the broader digital divide [7]. Although open-access publishing aims to make scientific information freely available, high article-processing charges (APCs) and unclear waiver policies can unintentionally reinforce global inequities, particularly limiting researchers and institutions in underserved communities from publishing and benefiting fully from open access.

5.4 New Directions in Open Science Publishing

The traditional model of article-processing charges (APCs) has faced criticism. There have also been calls for reform in the evolving landscape of open-access publishing. Some alternative models include institutional funding, partnerships such as SCOAP3, and diamond open access, in which neither authors nor readers pay fees. These models represent a shift towards more collective and transparent funding approaches for open-access publishing, addressing global inequities and financial burden on individual researchers.[7]. For example, a model called SciELO (Scientific Electronic Library Online). This model aims to promote open access to research articles and enhance the visibility of scientific publishing in Latin America, the Caribbean, Spain, and Portugal. SciELO is funded by participating members' governments and provides a centralized repository for free access to scholarly articles across various disciplines, including health sciences, social sciences, and humanities [8].

Recent years brought new movements, such as the San Francisco Declaration on Research Assessment (DORA) and Plan S, which promote open access and advocate for a change in the way that research is assessed and disseminated. DORA calls for a reformed approach to research assessment that moves away from journal impact factors and emphasizes the quality and societal relevance of scientific work over publication metrics.

Plan S, led by the COAlition S [9], is an initiative that mandates immediate open access for all research funded by its signatory organizations. Among others: European Research Council (ERC), UK Research and Innovation (UKRI), Wellcome Trust, Bill and Melinda Gates Foundation, World Health Organization, European Commission, Dutch Research Council, Science Foundation Ireland, Australia: National Health and Medical Research Council, Swiss National Science Foundation, Agence Nationale de la recherche France [9]. The plan advocates for universal access to publicly funded research by rejecting the traditional subscription model and paywalls. Under Plan S, journals must be either fully open-access or comply with open-access policies, ensuring that scientific knowledge is accessible to all. In line with these principles, movements such as SciELO [8] illustrate a growing commitment to a more open, collaborative, and accessible future for science [10].

5.5 What Is Open Science

Open science makes scientific research, data, and dissemination accessible for all of society, from academic professionals to the general public. It involves publishing open research, advocating for open access, and facilitating the publication and communication of scientific knowledge, including research data. Open science aims to eliminate barriers to information sharing by ensuring that research output is freely available under open licenses, enabling easier access and further development of scientific discoveries.

Open Science emphasizes transparency, accessibility, and collaboration. With growing skepticism toward scientific findings and a decline in public confidence in science and scientists [11], the significance of open science becomes more important. Open science practices, by providing free access to research data and methodologies, facilitate independent result verification, which could help to combat dis- and misinformation, an issue that became particularly critical during the COVID-19 pandemic.

Still, further and better strategies are required to combat dis- and misinformation than focusing on open science practices alone. While open science is often promoted as a solution, critics may argue that it could lead to an oversimplification of the scientific process. Although data initiatives (i.e., FAIR) advocate for transparency and broad access, not all scientific research can or should be completely open. There are legitimate reasons for restricting access to certain datasets, due to issues like data privacy, intellectual property, sensitive information, and the potential for misinterpretation of complex data by the public. Yet, even restricted data can follow the FAIR principles [3].

5.6 How to Practice Open Science

The transition to open science starts with three essential practices: open registration, open access, and open data and code, described in Table 5.1.

Open registration: After the research idea, you must write two key documents: a research protocol and a data management plan (See Chap. 2).

5.7 The Research Protocol

As mentioned in Chap. 2, for health, dental, or medical research, a research protocol usually includes the following key components:

1. **Title**: A clear, concise title that reflects the nature of the study.
2. **Background and Rationale**: Explanation of the problem being studied, previous research, and the significance of the study to the field.
3. **Objectives**: Specific aims or hypotheses the research intends to test or explore.
4. **Study Design**: Description of the type of study (e.g., randomized controlled trial, observational study, case-control study) and the rationale for choosing this design.

Table 5.1 Critical practices

What	How	Why	Where
Open Registration	Share your rationale, hypothesis, and methodology before conducting your research	Registering research protocols and methodologies before conducting an experiment increases transparency and reduces publication bias.	osf.io/registries, clinicaltrials.gov, www.isrctn.com, clinicaltrialsregister.eu, Prospero (for systematic reviews)
Open-Access Publications	Choose to publish your research as open access. However, be aware that there may be Article-Processing Costs (APC) involved	Scientific works are published as freely accessible to the public, eliminating cost barriers or access restrictions.	medRxiv.org, open-access publications, institutional repositories
Open Data	Share your research data openly	Data should be as open as possible and as close as necessary. To ensure the quality and utility of your data, it should adhere to the FAIR (findable, accessible, interoperable, and reusable) principles. Additionally, open code should be provided, where possible, to enhance reproducibility and transparency in computational research.	Zenodo.org, Figshare, dryad, osf.io

5. **Methodology**:
   (a) **Population/Participants**: Criteria for including and excluding participants and the target population.
   (b) **Intervention(s)**: If applicable, a detailed description of the intervention (for clinical trials), including dosage, frequency, and duration.
   (c) **Data Collection Methods**: Techniques and tools used to collect data (e.g., surveys, physical examinations, laboratory tests).
   (d) **Variables**: Provide a definition of primary and secondary outcome measures and any other data to be collected.
   (e) **Guidelines**: Depending on the specific question and study design, it is essential to consult the most appropriate guideline from the EQUATOR Network to ensure all methodological items are presented. For example, CONSORT is used for clinical trials, PRISMA is used for systematic reviews, STROBE is used for observational studies, and STARD is used for diagnostic research.
6. **Sample Size Calculation**: Explanation the unit of analysis (sample, tooth, patient?) and how the sample size was determined, including any assumptions made and statistical methods used.

7. **Data Analysis Plan:** Description of the statistical tests and procedures used to analyze the data, including any software employed. This section should also specify how missing data, outliers, and potential confounding factors will be handled.
8. **Dissemination Strategies**: The protocol should also outline dissemination strategies for the results, such as presentations at conferences, reports in peer-reviewed journals or websites, social media, or press releases.

Where possible, every effort should be made to adhere to any EQUATOR guidelines, although we acknowledged that this may not be feasible for all types of research design. In any case, by adhering to the relevant EQUATOR Network guidelines, researchers ensure that their studies are designed and reported with transparency and rigor, enhancing the reliability and reproducibility of the results. In addition, the research protocol is required to apply for ethical approval if your research involves humans or animals, and for funding or grants.

This research protocol represents your first publication. You can submit it to a journal specializing in research protocols, such as BMC Oral Health or Trials for clinical trial protocols. Alternatively, consider a repository tailored to your study type, such as PROSPERO for systematic reviews, or ClinicalTrials.gov for clinical trials. Another viable option is to select a general scientific repository, such as the Open Science Foundation registry.

5.8 The Research Data Management Plant

The second document for publication that must be prepared is the Data Management Plan (DMP). You should consider that your research will generate data crucial for addressing your research question, and this data should be managed carefully to ensure its integrity, security, and accessibility. Establishing a comprehensive DMP is essential not only for promoting good research practices but also for meeting the requirements of funding agencies and ethical standards.

In drafting a DMP, researchers need to outline how data will be collected, organized, stored, and shared throughout the research process. This includes specifying the types of data that will be generated, the methods of data collection, and the tools or software that will be employed for data analysis. Additionally, the plan should detail procedures for ensuring data quality and integrity, which are critical for maintaining the integrity of the research findings.

Some may find this familiar, as it largely overlaps with ethics clearance proposals submitted to ethics committees. Both documents require careful consideration of how data will be handled in a manner that respects participant confidentiality and adheres to ethical guidelines. For example, just as ethics clearance proposals mandate the protection of sensitive information, a well-constructed DMP must outline measures taken to safeguard the data from unauthorized access or breeches. Additionally, it should articulate the processes for obtaining informed consent regarding data use and sharing, thereby ensuring that participants are fully aware of how their information will be utilized and stored.

Moreover, the DMP should address long-term data preservation strategies, indicating where and how data will be archived post-research to ensure future accessibility and usability. This is increasingly important in today's research landscape, where data sharing and reuse are encouraged to promote collaborative knowledge advancement.

In summary, creating a detailed DMP can serve several purposes: it can enhance the integrity of the research project, it aligns with ethical expectations and through its publication fosters a responsible and transparent research environment. Box 5.1 outlines the main elements of a DMP.

Box 5.1 Elements in a data management plan

The elements typically included in a DMP document are as follows:

1. **Data Collection**:
   (a) Description of the data to be collected or generated
   (b) Methods for data collection and generation
   (c) Standards and metadata to be applied
2. **Documentation and Metadata**:
   (a) Information needed for data interpretation ○ Standards used for documentation and metadata
3. **Ethics and Legal Compliance**:
   (a) Consideration of ethical issues
   (b) Compliance with legal requirements and standards
   (c) Data protection and confidentiality measures
4. **Data Storage and Backup**:
   (a) How and where data will be stored and backed up
   (b) Security measures to protect data
5. **Data Sharing and Access**:
   (a) How data will be shared with the wider community
   (b) Conditions under which data can be accessed
   (c) Licensing for data reuse
6. **Responsibilities and Resources**:
   (a) Roles and responsibilities for data management
   (b) Resources required for data management
7. **Data Preservation**:
   (a) Plans for archiving and preserving data
   (b) Duration of data retention
8. **Budget and Funding**:
   (a) Budget considerations for data management
   (b) Funding sources for ongoing data management activities

These elements ensure that research data is well-managed, accessible, and preserved for future use, following best practice and compliance requirements.

Online tools are now available to assist in creating a DMP. One of these tools is ARGOS. ARGOS offers step-by-step guidance, templates, and examples, simplifying the creation of DMPs that meet the standards of various funding agencies and institutions.

5.8.1 *FAIR Research Data*

In addition, a DMP will make it easier to share the data once it has been generated following the FAIR principles, which emphasize that data should be Findable, Accessible, Interoperable, and Reusable.

FAIR data principles are guidelines to improve the findability, accessibility, interoperability, and reusability of digital assets. These principles serve as a foundational framework for enabling data and metadata, this is the data about the data, to be discoverable and usable by humans and machines long after the research has concluded. Table 5.2 presents the core components of FAIR data [3].

These principles guide researchers in making their datasets easily discoverable and accessible to humans or machines, ensuring that data can be integrated with other datasets and appropriately reused under clear and accessible data use licenses. Adherence to the FAIR principles increases the visibility and usability of research data and enhances the integrity and reliability of scientific research by enabling the validation and reproducibility of results. Implementing these principles in the

Table 5.2 FAIR principles [12] (Adapted from Bezjak et al., 2018 [12]. Some modifications were made. https://doi.org/10.5281/zenodo.1212496, licensed under the terms of the Creative Commons Zero v1.0 Universal License (https://creativecommons.org/publicdomain/zero/1.0/deed.en))

Principle	Definition	Example of Compliance
Findable	Data should be easily located by both humans and computers, with clear metadata and a unique identifier.	Use Digital Object Identifiers (DOIs) and rich metadata descriptions in data repositories like Zenodo or Figshare.
Accessible	Once found, data should be accessible with clearly defined access conditions, open or restricted.	Data hosted on platforms requiring login for sensitive data, or open access for nonsensitive data.
Interoperable	Data should be presented in a format seamlessly integrated with other datasets.	Use of open data formats and schemas such as CSV, HTML, or JSON that align with community standards.
Reusable	Data should be well-documented and stored in trusted repositories to ensure they can be effectively reused in future research.	To clarify permissible uses of the data, licenses such as CC BY (which allows sharing and adaptation with attribution) or CC0 (which dedicates works to the public domain) should be assigned.

research data management plan promotes transparency, maximizes research impact, and contributes to a more efficient and collaborative scientific ecosystem.

One of the most important parts of these principles is data sharing and reuse, not only for humans but for machines. Machines must be able to find and use this data or any digital object relevant to research.

This will ensure that the data created today can be used long term.

Remember that:

- FAIR is a set of principles, not a standard.
- Not all data has to be made open. Data can be restricted and still be FAIR, as these principles can ensure that data remains organized and accessible for potential use by others [3].
- Keep in mind: "As Open as Possible, As Closed as Necessary."

5.9 Open Science in Action

To illustrate how to apply the principles of open science in practice, let's explore a real-world example. This study focused on investigating the oral health conditions of children in rural areas of southern Chile [13].

During the initial literature review in any topic, it is not uncommon to encounter fragmented evidence. In this case, the researchers discovered numerous reports on the prevalence of early childhood caries from various countries, but no comprehensive synthesis was available. This gap led them to undertake a systematic review, ensuring their research approach was methodically transparent and collaborative.

5.10 The Pre-registration

The researchers registered their research intent and methodology on PROSPERO, the international database for systematic review protocols.

Uribe S, Maldupa I. Worldwide prevalence of early childhood caries: a systematic review.PROSPERO. https://www.crd.york.ac.uk/prospero/display_record.php?RecordID=9578.

This PROSPERO registration for a systematic review on the global prevalence of early childhood caries. The registration, a key step in the review process, documents the intent, methodology, and search strategy, helping to maintain research integrity and avoid duplication in the field. This step was also vital for maintaining the integrity of the review and preventing duplicate efforts in the research community.

5.11 Data Management and Sharing

To manage the data in a transparent manner and to allow for collaborative work, the researchers created a shared online folder using the Open Science Framework (OSF):

Uribe SE, Maldupa I, Innes N. DATASET The Global Prevalence of Early Childhood Caries: A Systematic Review with meta-analysis. Identifier: DOI:10.17605/OSF.IO/K7ZUN.

The published dataset on OSF accompanying a systematic review allows researchers to access raw data, replicate findings, or explore new hypotheses related to the global prevalence of early childhood caries. The researchers collected data via a Google Form, which automatically stored information in a CSV file, ensuring that our data was accessible and in an open format. All subsequent analyses were conducted using R, an open-source statistical software, to promote the reproducibility and accessibility of the analytical methods used.

5.12 Sharing Our Findings in an Open-Access Publication

This is an example of a publication demonstrating open science practices through open-access publication, pre-registration, and open data availability: The researchers cited the OSF repository that housed the raw data in their final open-access publication. This citation ensured compliance with open science practices and was a resource for further independent analysis. It also enabled the broader scientific community to scrutinize the methodologies used. The article includes sections like "Materials and Methods" and a "Data Availability Statement," highlighting open science practices, including protocol registration, open data access, and analysis script [13]:

Uribe SE, Innes N, Maldupa I. The global prevalence of early childhood caries: A systematic review with meta-analysis using the WHO diagnostic criteria. Int J Paediatr Dent. 2021;31:817-830. doi: 10.1111/ipd.12783.

This case study exemplifies the application of open science principles, demonstrating how researchers can manage, share, and disseminate their findings to foster a more collaborative, transparent, and accessible scientific landscape.

Adhering to open science, particularly in data management strategies, saved us time and provided a reusable framework. Even now, the researchers often refer to portions of the code used in the original research for new projects. Furthermore, they designed this research with future updates in mind, anticipating that new researchers can easily add updated data every 10 years and reanalyze the findings. This approach extends the lifespan and utility of the work and significantly increases its impact, as ongoing updates will keep the research relevant and continually integrated into newer scientific developments.

5.13 Conclusion

The publication of findings remains central to scientific activity. However, it is also important that new knowledge is not confined to the walls of libraries but shared among others, allowing anybody to build upon and refine these findings. The chapter advocates for the adoption of open protocols, which not only promote transparency but facilitate the replication of studies. The importance of this replicability cannot be overstated. When researchers share their methodologies openly, they empower others to verify their results, challenge assumptions, and ultimately contribute to a more robust and reliable body of knowledge. Furthermore, this chapter stressed the significance of publishing in open-access journals. Open-access publishing removes the barriers, financial or otherwise, that often restrict access to scientific information. Finally, sharing the collected data, ideally following the FAIR principles, enables others to replicate and validate the findings, as well as explore new hypotheses, thereby increasing the impact of the original research.

References

1. Rabba JA, Efenji GI, Uloko FO, Amuda DB, Jaafar HA, Suhaimi FM, Osman ND. Investigation of the optimal tube voltage kV exposure parameters for general X-ray of dental cone-beam computed tomography: a cephalometric view. Adv Radiother Nucl Med. 2024;2:2972.
2. Riaud X. First dental radiograph (1896). Dent Hist. 2014;59:87–8.
3. National Institute for Open Science (NIOS). Everyone wants to play FAIR, but what does that really mean? 2024. https://ni4os.eu/2020/02/07/everyone-wants-to-play-fair-but-what-does-that-really-mean/# Accessed 15 November 2024.
4. Nejstgaard CH, Laursen DRT, Lundh A, Hróbjartsson A. Commercial funding and estimated intervention effects in randomized clinical trials: Systematic review of meta-epidemiological studies. Res Synth Methods. 2023;14:144–55.
5. Australian Government. NHMRC Open Access Policy. 2023. https://www.nhmrc.gov.au/aboutus/resources/nhmrc-open-access-policy. Accessed 13 November 2024.
6. Ellis RJ. Questionable Research Practices, Low Statistical Power, and Other Obstacles to Replicability: Why Preclinical Neuroscience Research Would Benefit from Registered Reports. eNeuro. 2022;9:ENEURO.0017-22.2022. doi: 10.1523/ENEURO.0017-22.2022.
7. Sanderson K. Who should pay for open-access publishing? APC alternatives emerge Nature. 2023;623(7987):472–3. https://doi.org/10.1038/d41586-023-03506-4.
8. Scientific Electronic Library Online (Scielo). https://scielo.org/en/. Accessed 18 November 2024.
9. Plan S. Organizations endorsing Plan S and working jointly on its implementation. 2024. https://www.coalition-s.org/organisations/ Accessed 15 November 2024.
10. Cole NL, Kormann E, Klebel T, Apartis S, Ross-Hellauer T. The societal impact of Open Science: a scoping review. R Soc Open Sci. 2024;11:240286. https://doi.org/10.1098/rsos.240286.
11. Lupia A, Allison DB, Jamieson KH, Heimberg J, Skipper M, Wolf SM. Trends in U.S. public confidence in science and opportunities for progress. Proc Natl Acad Sci USA. 2024;121(11):e2319488121. https://doi.org/10.1073/pnas.2319488121.

12. Bezjak S, Clyburne-Sherin A, Conzett P, Fernandes P, Görögh E, Helbig K, Kramer B, Labastida I, Niemeyer K, Psomopoulos F, Ross-Hellauer T, Schneider R, Tennant J, Verbakel E, Brinken H, Heller L. Open Science Training Handbook (1.0) [Computer software]. Zenodo; 2018. https://doi.org/10.5281/zenodo.1212496. Accessed 29 April 2025.
13. Uribe SE, Innes N, Maldupa I. The global prevalence of early childhood caries: a systematic review with meta-analysis using the WHO diagnostic criteria. Int J Paediatr Dent. 2021;31:817–30. https://doi.org/10.1111/ipd.12783.

Chapter 6
Preparation of an Original Article: Writing the Introduction

Rodrigo Mariño

6.1 Introduction

As mentioned in Chaps. 2 and 5, there are many ways to publish research. This manual will generally focus on scientific journal articles, but many of the aspects that will be discussed are useful for other forms of publication. In those chapters, it was mentioned that there may be different documents that are related to the same study: a study protocol, a thesis, and a manuscript. All of which have different formats, but they all have an introduction. The same applies to abstracts or posters, another way of publishing at a conference, and oral presentations (See Chap. 12). All formats have an introduction, a title of course, and, usually, an abstract.

Therefore, the objective of this chapter is to describe the different components of a scientific publication, describing in detail the title and the introduction. It will describe the importance of the introduction, what its components are, and the elements that an introduction should have. It will also cover aspects of the title page, which is another document that many scientific journals ask for when submitting a manuscript for review. However, the focus of the chapter will be the introduction itself.

R. Mariño (✉)
Melbourne Dental School, The University of Melbourne, Melbourne, Australia

Center for Research in Epidemiology, Economics and Oral Public Health (CIEESPO), University de la Frontera, Temuco, Chile

Department of Conservative Dentistry and Oral Health, Riga Stradins University, Riga, Latvia

Monash Health Dental Services, Melbourne, Australia
e-mail: r.marino@unimelb.edu.au

R. Mariño et al. (eds.), *Scientific Writing and Publication Strategies for Oral Health Professionals*, https://doi.org/10.1007/978-3-031-97916-3_6

6.2 Familiarize with the Target Journal Format

Once the target journal has been selected, which will be the topic of Chap. 11, the first thing to do, and this also applies for the whole manuscript preparation, is to become familiar with the format of the journal. To do this, you must read the instructions for authors. After you have read the authors' instructions, read them, and re-read them again. The objective is that you become familiar with all the details and everything that is being asked for the submission of the manuscript.

Follow the manuscript format to the letter (See Box 6.1). If this is not done, the manuscript will return within a few hours of being submitted. This is the first filter applied to the manuscript by an administrative officer who checks that all requirements have been met. This is not a scientific review of the quality of the manuscript, but merely a formatting one. However, it is very important because if it is not formatted and submitted as requested, although it may not be rejected at this stage, the manuscript will be returned to you so that you can format it following the journal requirements.

Some author guidelines have several pages detailing the steps to follow. So, the time spent reading and becoming familiar with the information in the journal being targeted for submission is very important. It is an investment.

Of course, in some cases you do not have to follow all the guidelines because there will be items that do not apply to your specific manuscript. This depends on whether it is an editor's letter, a case report, a literature review, etc. In each case there will be different guidelines. Once you identify the type of manuscript you are submitting, follow these steps rigorously.

Box 6.1 Journal's format
Get familiar with the Journal's format

- Read the instructions for authors
- Re-read and re-read the instructions …!!
- Follow manuscript format
  - Word limit
  - Margins
  - Fonts: type and size
  - Page numbering style and place.
  - Is compliance with any standards required? For example, trial reports ("CONSORT").
  - How references are to be cited

All these small details, as mentioned, have absolutely nothing to do with the scientific quality of the manuscript, but you must follow them because if not the manuscript will be returned to you before even going to peer review.

Once you are familiar with the format, note the word limit, what the margins are, the type and size of the fonts requested, the number of pages and include page numbers, if requested, in the correct location, i.e. at the bottom of the page or at the top.

Depending on the type of study, compliance with an existing standard may be required, for example, CONSORT for clinical trials. How references are to be cited is also important, and this is all stated in the instructions to the author. Therefore, read it and follow it as closely and correctly as possible.

6.3 How Is Manuscript Writing Done?

As we mentioned earlier, writing a manuscript is a slow, complicated, and iterative process. And it is such because we must summarize 2 or 3 years of work in a few thousand words (e.g., 3000–3500), which may require certain training and skills. This writing is usually done in a group. Thus, it is important that all those recognized as authors or co-authors actively participate in the process.

It might be worthwhile to have a look at other manuscripts that have been published in the target journal to get an idea of their format. However, use caution as sometimes the manuscript published in a journal will not follow the same format as the one requested for peer review.

Look at a published manuscript for style, but always refer to the guidelines for authors to follow the steps.

Preparing a manuscript to be submitted takes time. Once all authors and co-authors are satisfied with its content, we begin the process of preparing the manuscript to be submitted for peer-review, which is also time-consuming and frustrating. One may wonder: why do I have to do it this way when it has nothing to do with the scientific quality of my manuscript? However, those are the rules.

What can happen is that in many cases authors do not continue this process once they have already started preparing the paper. So, if things are out of order from the beginning, the time required of the journal's editors and reviewers, who are generally volunteers, will be wasted. So, follow all the steps and review all documents available.

If you are going to use the CONSORT [1] or another reporting guideline [2], you may need to declare it (i.e., "*This publication follows the guide of CONSORT,*" STROBE, or other applicable guideline). You may also be asked to provide the corresponding checklist as part of the submission. Additionally, following the guide makes it easier for you to organize the material and write the manuscript.

If possible, seek mentors or consult with researchers who have more experience in publishing and always look at the clarity of the descriptions.

6.4 The Elements of a Manuscript

The main elements of a manuscript are the title, abstract, introduction, methodology, results, and discussion. It is suggested that the title and abstract are usually written last. Of course, you can start with a tentative title, but at the end of writing the manuscript you must revise and finish it (See Box 6.2).

The abstract comes from the manuscript itself. Many journals use the IMRAD structure, which is Introduction, Methodology, Results, and Discussion. That is the general format but as mentioned, not all journals share this. For example, there are some that ask for a conclusion section to be separate from the discussion.

6.4.1 The Title

The title, as already mentioned, may not be the first thing that is written, it may even be the last. The title is a mini summary of the study. The title should capture the essence and accurately represent the content of the study, or the manuscript. Keep in mind that when you do a literature review, the first thing you will see is the titles of the references. Based on the title, you are going to decide whether you will continue reading the manuscript or not. Therefore, it is very important.

Box 6.2 The elements of a manuscript
The elements of a manuscript

- **Title**: Concise and effective
- Abstract
  - IMRaD
- **Introduction** (Clear, easy to understand, convincing)
  - Rational
  - Literature
  - Significance
  - Outline objectives
- **Methodology**
- **Results**
- **Discussion**

The title should not be ambiguous, it must be clear and easily understood on the first reading. Avoid titles that look or sound good or use compelling language purely aimed at attention- grabbing. This is not a newspaper story. The title of a newspaper article always tries to attract attention with what is said, but yours is a scientific publication, not show business or for word games. Additionally, this may put off some reviewers if it is not their style. Therefore, try to give off a good initial impression to the reader or reviewer regarding the content of the study.

Remember that in some journals, one of the guidelines includes a word or character limit for the title. It should generally be no longer than 10 or 15 words. It must be precise, using terms that accurately reflect what is to be studied or what was studied. It must be simple; written in the language we use daily at our professional level. It may also contain or give an outline of the design of the study and the population to be studied.

To do this, review the publications in a journal that you consider prestigious or in which you want to publish for ideas on how to generate titles. Remember that there is a common title for a series of documents, including proposals for research funding.

According to Ecarnot and collaborators [3], these are elements to include in a title:

- ***Name the factors studied*** (or to be studied). For example, what type of intervention is going to be conducted, or what type of maneuver is going to be performed, what drug is going to be used, etc.
- ***Name the population studied***, or the context of the study. For example, in patients with myocardial infarction.
- ***Name the study design***. Cohort study, cross-sectional, randomized clinical trial, etc.
- ***Cite most important findings***. Increases, reduces, prevents, etc.
- ***Include the most important aspect first***. It is what distinguishes the manuscript from other studies.
- ***Avoid being imprecise.***

Here is an example of a title:

"Periodontitis as a risk factor for myocardial infarction; A case-control study" [4].

This is a clear title, indicating what was studied, the disease or condition in focus, and the study design. It does not describe the population, but it is clear and hints at what the content of the article will be [3, 4].

It has also become fashionable to use acronyms to name a study. You may or may not use them, it is not necessary, but it has become fashionable in recent years.

There are times when the title has two parts separated by a colon, a general part and a slightly more specific part. This is also something that you should consider. There are some journals that advise against this, and of course, there are reviewers who may not like this style.

Jacques et al. describe the importance of the title and mention some techniques for how to make the title appear in searches. They conclude, after conducting a review, that the construction of the manuscript's title has an impact on the frequency with which the article is cited [5].

Therefore, the title, although it has 10 or 15 words, will produce an effect on the impact of the scientific production that you may have. Consequently, we must award it the importance it deserves.

6.5 How to Write an Introduction

The introduction must be clear, easy to understand, convincing, follow a rationale, be based on literature, indicate significance, and outline the objectives of the study. This section is important because you must attract the reader's attention and capture their interest to continue reading the manuscript. Box 6.3 presents the main elements of an introduction section.

The introduction should provide answers to two questions:

- What is going to be done? and
- For what purpose?

Many times, and you may have experienced this yourself, once we have read the introduction we do not continue reading. This might be because the manuscript is not relevant to the topic of your search, but it may also be because the introduction does not create any incentive to continue reading the manuscript. On the contrary, the aim is that when the audience reads the introduction, they think: "*why this good idea did not occur to me?*".

The introduction must contain the formulation of the problem, its importance, and the scope and level of research. It includes a brief but critical review of the literature; what is known about the problem, what is unknown, and the gap that is going to be filled with the study to be presented. It must also contain general and specific objectives, and if the design is appropriate, the hypotheses to be tested.

Box 6.3 The elements of an introduction
The introduction section must minimally contain:

- Formulation of the problem
- Importance and scope of the research
- Critical review of the literature
  - What is known about the problem?
  - What is not known
  - The gap to be filled
- General and specific objectives
- Hypothesis (in analytical designs)

There are different styles, and some suggest stating the objectives within the methodology. I believe that the reader should know as soon as possible what the study is about. However, this is a matter of styles or guidelines to the authors. Likewise, there are those who say that the hypothesis should come before the objectives, others say that the objectives first and then the hypotheses, again this is a matter of style.

6.5.1 *Formulation of the Problem and the Importance of the Research*

To formulate the problem, you must briefly state what is going to be solved, what the topic is, but only very briefly. Start at a general level and go to the more specific, ensuring that the importance of the problem emanates from its formulation.

The importance of the question to be investigated must be highlighted, demonstrating that it has not been answered before and that this proposed work will answer it. You can, although this might also be part of the methodology, mention the theoretical model that will be used. If included in the introduction, it then can be expanded in the methodology. However, the significance must be pointed out: for what or whom these results can be used; for public policies, or to improve a type of care, to improve patient quality of life, etc. A couple of sentences in this regard can be included.

The significance and relevance of the research question is crucial because reviewers will be looking for it. In many cases, the authors present descriptions of the work: "Study of 200 cases of implants in University of Lake Wobegon dental clinic." This is very relevant at the local level and may be for audit purposes, but think from an international perspective: what new information or knowledge is being provided? If the results only have local significance and the manuscript does not offer a new vision that goes beyond this environment, it has less chance of being accepted in an international journal. Studies can have strong local relevance, but the authors need to demonstrate and emphasize its international significance.

When demonstrating the importance of what is going to be studied, its applicability and utility should be highlighted through practical application: "The study is responding to the national oral health plan"; "to the requirements of the country's health plan"; "The study is responding to requirements for new health policies," etc. The issue must be positioned within a larger context and have national or international importance and relevance.

When writing the introduction of a scientific paper, a common mistake is assuming that the absence of research or reviews in a specific area justifies new research. For instance, while numerous studies may explore the association between maternal smoking and dental caries in children, the lack of a systematic review on this topic does not necessarily indicate the need for one. Prior research consistently confirms this association, and a new review may not add meaningful insights to the existing body of knowledge.

This approach represents a weak foundation for justifying research, as it is essential to ensure that the study genuinely addresses a gap in the literature rather than simply reiterating established knowledge.

6.5.2 *Critical Review of the Literature*

This chapter will not go into detail about how to critically review literature, or on how to do searches. You should already have some experience in this area. Nonetheless, the introduction should briefly synthesize and critically analyze the most relevant works to the topic under study. The introduction must support and provide evidence of what is being demonstrated or argued. Perhaps the keywords here are *synthesize* and *critical analysis*. The purpose of the literature review in the introduction section is to provide the theoretical foundation for the work to be carried out.

Box 6.4 Purpose of the literature review
Purpose of the literature review

- Verify the relevance of the problem to be studied
- Define the problem to be investigated
- Need and rationale for the study
- Identify key areas that need to be investigated
- Establish the theoretical basis of the problem
- Identify the research design
- Identify measurement instruments
- Identify strategies for data analysis
- Put conclusions into perspective

I personally, to use a sport term, am a fan of literature reviews. I believe that a good literature review will significantly enable the work ahead for a study. A good review will tell us what needs to be done, because it will provide an indication of the as-yet unknown aspects, what part of the problem we should focus on, and which methodology to use. Later, in the discussion section, it will help us place our work and results within the context of the literature.

The first four points in Box 6.4 are part of the introduction section. For the introduction, we must highlight the relevance of the problem, indicate which part of the issue to be investigated has not been studied before, or if it was, the missing elements, or those that are unclear or controversial and must therefore be answered through our study. This will help us support the study and provide it with rationale and significance. All of this is part of the introduction.

When considering the methods section, the literature review will help us establish the theoretical framework of the problem, identify the research design, the instruments that we will use to collect the data, and strategies for data analysis. It is possible that each section of the manuscript will require different literature reviews.

The role of the literature review in the introduction is:

- To **reflect** on the material
- To **synthesize** the information
- To demonstrate that you have **current** information on the topic
- To demonstrate that you manage information **coherently**
- Provide the arguments to rigorously demonstrate that the research is effectively addressing existing **gaps** in our knowledge.

The literature review is an iterative process, which must be repeated several times and perhaps, as mentioned above, with different objectives. The bad news is that a literature review must be done to the end, "*all the way,*" as Frank Sinatra sang. This cannot be ignored. On the other hand, the good news is that most of the time you have a deadline, and it must end at some point. What you can do is conduct an initial review, write the paper and maybe when you are ready to submit the manuscript, conduct another review to make sure there are no new publications in the area.

Consider that the process of writing a manuscript may take several weeks, even months. There may be something published in that period that is relevant to the topic we are working on, and the peer review will be done by experts on the subject. Therefore, you might identify that some current references on that topic are missing. So do a quick check in case, more so if it is a thesis or a 2–3-year research project, because in that long period new material may well have been published on the subject.

6.6 How to Catch Beginners? [6]

Lack of integration. The paragraphs and information are not integrated and there is a lack of a logical structure for describing literature. For example, "Smiths and collaborators say…", then in another separate paragraph, "Jones indicates…", "Rodríguez, his collaborators conclude …". These three paragraphs are not linked and there is no integration of the information, no natural flow of ideas and arguments. It is written as a summary of literature. The paragraphs are descriptive only, when all of this can be within the same topic or section.

This lack of integration may be present within the introduction, but it may also be missing across the entire document. This must be avoided, and an effort must be made to integrate the information that exists in the literature and make reading easier. Hence the need to work with colleagues to improve writing.

Does not demonstrate good knowledge of the aspects of this research. Remember that the manuscript or a thesis will be reviewed by experts on the subject. They are likely to be aware and knowledgeable of the literature and identify whether the authors did not review recent literature or the lack of important or recent references on the topic.

Avoid secondary references. This occurs when the authors of a manuscript include a reference for information that is not the original, primary source. For example, health is defined as: "*A state of complete physical, mental and social well-being, and not merely the absence of disease*" [7], a quote from the World Health Organization (WHO) that is widely used. Therefore, if you use that definition, cite the WHO and not cite an author who used it, that is, a secondary reference. Always go to the original source.

In some cases, there may be seminal works on the topic of the proposed study, which was published 50, 60, or more years ago. This work must be acknowledged as the beginning of a line of research. You can acknowledge this, but, in general, you must ***use recent references.***

Especially, one of the most common failures is ***not thinking critically.*** Always question the information. Do not accept something as correct just because it was published. It may not be up to date and the information may be incomplete or contain errors, etc.

Therefore, it is important to always question and critically appraise what we read. When you review an article, you should ascertain:

- How convincing and valid the evidence is,
- Whether the findings are consistent with other studies,
- How generalizable are the findings?

There are findings that are particularly specific to some populations. In this case, identify the population for which it is most relevant. This is about being critical of the information and again, if valid evidence is provided, are there alternative explanations for the results, from what you know, or from the literature?

Rudyard Kipling wrote: "*I keep six honest serving-men (They taught me all I knew); Their names are What and Why and When and How and Where and Who*" [8]. The literature review section of the introduction should answer these questions succinctly but comprehensively. Interpretation is important, but one must be critical.

When writing the literature review, there might be some definitions and terms to be clarified for the reader. However, although that will depend on the topic, those terms do not always need to be explained in detail. It depends on which journal the manuscript is to be sent to. If it is a dental journal, for example, it is likely that explanations of the indices used do not require extensive explanations because they will be well understood. When an oral health manuscript is submitted to a non-dental journal, these may need to be explained. However, there are always examples which are considered common knowledge and do not need to be explained in detail.

In summary, the important thing is that you begin writing your introduction section document. When you start the introduction, write and write. The manuscripts to be sent for publication will have some 3000–3500 words, but when you start do not worry about word limits, just write. You can "*prune*" the writing as you progress in preparing the manuscript.

When writing the introduction of a scientific paper, one common mistake is assuming that the absence of research or reviews in a specific area justifies new research. For instance, while numerous studies may explore the association between maternal smoking and dental caries in children, there needs to be a systematic review on this topic to signal the need for one. A new review might not add meaningful insight if prior research consistently confirms the association. This approach represents a weak foundation for justifying the research, as it is crucial to ensure that the study addresses a genuine gap in the literature rather than simply restating established knowledge.

6.7 Purpose and Objectives

The purpose gives a general direction to what we want to study. The objectives, on the other hand, define more precisely what is going to be measured. The purpose is usually unique and captures the essence of the study in a sentence or paragraph [9]. That paragraph should provide a synopsis of the purpose of the study. In scientific articles, it is usually found at the end of the introduction, but in longer publications such as a report, a book or a thesis, the purpose may form a separate chapter.

A statement of the purpose of a study should include:

1. The central concept to be studied
2. The unit of analysis (person, group, place, anatomical area, organ, etc.)
3. The methodology used for data collection
4. Terms that would not be easily understood by the reader (Note: this is different from our description of variables that we will see in Chap. 7).

The objectives refer to the aspects that you want to study or the immediate results that you hope to obtain to answer the final problem. The objectives define with greater precision the aspects that are going to be studied; they are formulated in relation to the problem being studied and its purpose. The objectives have several goals [10]. These are:

1. To guide the study
2. Determine the limits of the study
3. Provide guidance on the results expected to be obtained
4. Allow the stages of the study to be established

The formulation of objectives is done following certain criteria. The objectives are generally written in the infinitive tense and must:

1. Be directed to the basic elements of the problem
2. Be measurable and observable
3. Be clear and precise
4. Follow a methodological order

Therefore, the objectives will guide us on our path. If we do not have a goal, we will certainly get somewhere, but it may not be where we wanted.

The dialogue below is taken from Lewis Carroll's famous novel, "Alice's Adventures in Wonderland." It represents a conversation between Alice and the Cheshire Cat. This dialogue highlights the importance of having a clear objective or destination in mind when making decisions or choosing a path. Without a goal, the choices we make may lack purpose or direction.

> *"Alice: Would you tell me, please, which way I ought to go from here? The Cheshire Cat: That depends a good deal on where you want to get to.*
> *Alice: I don't much care where.*
> *The Cheshire Cat: Then it doesn't much matter which way you go"*
> —Lewis Carroll, Alice in Wonderland [11].

My personal preference is to place the purpose and objective early in the manuscript, where appropriate, in the introduction section. Once we have demonstrated that there is a lack of knowledge in the literature, we can show that our study answers it by generating our objectives.

6.7.1 How to Create Objectives

The research question will, or should, lead us in a logical way to the design of the purpose and objectives of the study. The objectives must indicate what you want to achieve, how it will be achieved, and who the beneficiaries are. The general objective of the study must be generated from the research question. So, ask yourself:

- What am I trying to achieve? and write that in a few words.
- How am I going to achieve this?

From there, an initial indication of purpose and objective must be generated. An objective must be clear, but not necessarily very sophisticated, and understandable to a professionally educated person.

There may be a general objective and one or more specific objectives. The general objectives specify the phenomenon or intervention in a broad way, which population we want to study, etc.

The specific objectives are more detailed: what we want to study once we have identified the variables to be measured and that we want to describe.

An objective must be measurable, observable, achievable, concrete, logical, and relevant. For these purposes, the SMART criteria are widely used for setting objectives in various fields. "SMART" is an acronym that stands for Specific, Measurable, Achievable, Relevant, and Time-bound goals. Using the SMART criteria can significantly enhance your ability to achieve them and provides a clearer roadmap for personal and professional development [12].

Let's consider an example that encompasses all aspects of the SMART framework:

Objective: I want to publish a manuscript in a high-impact dental public journal (Specific) and work with my data 1 h every day (Achievable) for the next 3 months with the goal of completing the manuscript in less than 4000 words (Measurable) by December 31st of this year (Time-bound).

Moreover, in the objectives section you can identify where the study is going to be carried out. This will depend on the focus and objectives of the research. For example, if the study focuses on the evaluation of a new dental treatment, it will likely be conducted in a clinical setting or a laboratory, where appropriate testing and analysis can be conducted. In other cases, such as in epidemiological studies, research may be carried out by collecting data in specific communities or populations. In addition, there are *in-situ* studies and *in-vivo* studies. Therefore, determining where the study will be conducted will depend on multiple factors, such as the research design, the availability of resources, and the nature of the phenomenon being studied.

Each specific objective will have an individual design and methodology leading to individual results and conclusions. While these are individual elements, they can also be viewed within the larger context. At some point you must put together those specific objectives into one study, which will be in the conclusion section of the discussion.

Table 6.1 presents an example of SMART objectives.

Table 6.1 Example of SMART objectives

Criteria	Good SMART Objective	Bad SMART Objective
Specific	To evaluate the effectiveness of fluoride varnish treatment in reducing dental caries in school-aged children (ages 6–12) in a low- income community.	To study fluoride and their effects on children's oral health
Measurable	The reduction of caries incidence will be measured by the number of new carious lesions identified in dental exams before and 6 months after the intervention.	Effect on caries
Achievable	The study will enroll 200 children from three schools in the community, with biannual application of fluoride varnish.	Not mentioned
Relevant	Fluoride varnish is a proven intervention, and this study will provide important data to support preventive dental care in low- income areas.	Not mentioned or supported by relevant references
Time-bound	The study will be conducted over a 12- month period, with baseline and follow-up dental exams at 6 months.	No timeframe mentioned.
Objective	To assess the effectiveness of fluoride varnish in reducing the incidence of dental caries among 200 school-aged children (6–12 years) in a low-income community over a 12-month period.	To study the effects of fluoride on children caries.

For example, we want to compare the height of male and female students in the last year of the Doctor in Dental Surgery at the University of Lake Wobegon, in 2024. This is our purpose. The objective would be to know the heights of women, to know the heights of men, and to compare the average heights of men and women. Those are our specific objectives. We can also state what tests we are going to use, but this may not be as necessary.

So, the purpose we had was to measure and compare the height of men and women. We can also generate a hypothesis. Our hypothesis would be that men will have a greater average height than women. This is based on the literature. We reviewed the literature about the topic and our conclusion was that, in general, men of the same age have a greater average height. That is a hypothesis that can be tested. See Box 6.5 for examples of a purpose and an objective.

Box 6.5 Example of purpose and objectives
Example

Purpose: what you plan to do

To compare the height of men and women in the last year of the dentistry degree at the University of Lake Wobegon, 2024.

Objective: how you plan to do it

1. To know the height of female students.
2. To know the height of male students.
3. To compare the means of men and women (using a t test)

6.8 The Hypothesis

A hypothesis is an assumption that establishes relationships between facts. The value of a hypothesis lies in its ability to establish these relationships and explain why they occur [10]. Thus, hypotheses are tentative statements of a relationship between at least two variables. Hypotheses are "educated" guesses about the relationships between these variables and the results of the study.

Hypotheses are constructs that guide the direction of the study. A hypothesis has five essential characteristics [10]. First, it must contain an independent variable, which is one that is believed to cause an effect on another variable, known as the dependent variable. Secondly, there must be a relationship between these variables, that is, the independent variable is expected to have some type of impact or influence on the dependent variable. Third, the hypothesis must include a clear and specific prediction about the direction or nature of this relationship. Fourth, the hypothesis must be based on existing theories or relevant prior information, thus supporting its logical foundation. Finally, the hypothesis must be feasible and capable of being tested through data collection and analysis. If a hypothesis cannot be confirmed or denied through empirical evidence, it does not meet the criteria of a valid hypothesis (See Box 6.6).

Some authors prefer to present the hypotheses before the objectives, while others choose to place them after. This depends on the researcher's style and preference. There are studies that do not test hypotheses but rather generate them, as is the case with descriptive studies. In descriptive studies, the hypotheses are usually implicit.

Box 6.6 The hypothesis

A **hypothesis** has five characteristics [10]:

1. Contains at least **one independent variable** and at least **one dependent variable**
2. Expresses **a relationship** between variables
3. Must be **a prediction**
4. Must be **based on theory** and what is known about a phenomenon, and
5. It must be **verifiable**

Now, this might seem a bit abstract, but it is not so in reality. We put hypotheses to the test every day, without even noticing. Here is an example: we tried to turn on the computer and it will not work. That is the problem. What do we do? We generate hypotheses about it and put them to the test:

Hypothesis 1) I pressed the wrong button. I verify that hypothesis and verify that, in fact, the button was the right one.

Hypothesis 2) The computer is out of charge/unplugged. I verify those hypotheses and verify that the computer either has a charge or it is plugged in.

Hypothesis 3) The cables are not connected. Other hypotheses that I can verify.

Hypothesis 4) I did not pay the electricity bill, they cut off my electricity.

Hypothesis 5) There is a blackout in the neighborhood.

Sometimes hypotheses can be statistical, such as a null hypothesis and the alternative hypothesis. You may have worked on them when learning statistical analysis. However, these are working hypotheses. They will usually not be part of the manuscript and are established to verify if there is any statistically significant effect or relationship between the variables under study.

Use the appropriate verb to measure, to evaluate, to analyze, to differentiate, to compare, to examine, to enumerate, etc. that fits the purpose and objective of the study you are doing. Next formulate the hypothesis. Keep in mind that the hypothesis is based on evidence from the literature. That is what needs to be structured in the introduction.

Focus the knowledge of the discipline on the research question you have, what you know about the topic on the research question, and state why that question is important. That is, for you as authors it is important, but you must consider the reader. Why is it important for them?

Table 6.2 Example of introduction writing

Purpose	Example
Describe the current state of knowledge:	"Dental caries is a common disease in the population"
Describe what other authors have observed/published:	"Cabrera et al. (2020) demonstrated that Fluoride solution A reduces the incidence of dental caries, while solution B does not do so."
Describe the process that has already started, but has not yet been completed:	"Many researchers have studied the effect of Fluoride A solution on dental caries"
Describe what has not yet been determined:	"It has not yet been determined whether…"
Formulate your goals:	This study has the purpose/objective of (measure, etc.) …
Formulate your hypotheses:	Fluoride A solution will reduce the incidence of caries in the population P in a XX%

In summary, the introduction describes the current state of knowledge. As an example, research on the effect of fluoride solution on dental caries has been widely studied, however, there are still gaps in knowledge. See Table 6.2 for an example of how to write an introduction.

You must also provide the necessary background and information, but at the same time, be brief. It is possible that the reader is already familiar with the topic but as mentioned, that would depend on the audience. However, keep in mind the minimum required information that a reader should have on the topic.

The literature review in the introduction may not provide all the details but remember that most of the literature that you would review might be relevant to other sections of the manuscript, for example, the discussion or even the methodology sections.

Remember that each sentence in the introduction must have a purpose. This is important in view of the word limit. Therefore, you must calculate and create a budget for how many words you need and determine where you can include more or less for the manuscript and introduction.

This is not a golden rule, and you will not find it written anywhere, but consider that the introduction should be 10 to 15% of the total words. If it is 3500 words, therefore, the introduction will be 350 to 500 words. Within those 350–500 words, you must include the research topic, or problem statement, the study's rationale, the research questions, and aims and objectives. Therefore, it is important to be brief and review the need for the information you provide.

The topic is specified, a justification for its importance is presented, the research question is formulated, a gap in current knowledge is demonstrated, and the purpose of the study is delineated along with the objectives of the study. This is a summary of the structure of our introduction, which should be between 350 and 500 words. It should also have a natural and coherent flow. As mentioned, by the end of the introduction, it should be evident to the reader that this topic needs to be studied.

6.9 Title Page

Some journals ask for a title page separate from the main part of the manuscript. This is because, for the review to be blind, it must be separate from its manuscript as the names, affiliations, and contacts of the authors will appear in the title page. Again, you should verify what each journal asks for. Some journals ask for the author's last name and initial, others for the first and last name and affiliation. Others ask for titles, position, etc. Other journals ask to include the ORCID number of the authors. The important thing is that the guidelines are reviewed and followed to the letter.

Be aware that authorship is only attributed when a researcher has made a significant intellectual or academic contribution to the manuscript and must take responsibility for some part of the study or manuscript. If not, authorship may be questioned.

Generally, a corresponding author is added on the title page and there is also a detailed format for how to introduce the corresponding author. This should all be described in the guidelines for authors.

You may be asked to include keywords on the title page. These keywords are generated from identifiers used by the National Library of Medicine. Authors can select those that apply for their specific manuscript [13]. Among other things, they serve to identify the reviewers.

Appendix

Activity 6.1
1) Describe the project you are interested in working on. Write your answer here: ____________________ ____________________ ____________________
2) For the selected project, write the background section - what is currently known about the topic and what is yet to be discovered (2 or 3 paragraphs): Write your answer here: ____________________ ____________________ ____________________
2.1) Describe the current state of knowledge. For example, "Dental caries is a common disease in the population": Write your answer here: ____________________ ____________________ ____________________
2.2) Describe what has been observed/published by other authors. For example, "Cabrera et al. (2020) demonstrated that Fluoride solution A reduces the incidence of cavities, however, solution B does not": Write your answer here: ____________________ ____________________ ____________________
2.3) Describe past research that still requires investigation. For example, "Many researchers have studied the effect of Fluoride A solution on dental caries": Write your answer here: ____________________ ____________________ ____________________
2.4) Describe what is still undetermined. For example, "It has yet to be determined if…": Write your answer here: ____________________ ____________________ ____________________
3) Write your specific Research Question. If you think there is more than one research question, write them all down. If you think there is more than one way to phrase your research questions, write all these down, too.

(*continued*)

(continued)

<table>
<tr><td>Write your answer here: ____
____
____</td></tr>
<tr><td>4) Indicate the significance of your project, the "So what?". Why is the study necessary? Indicate the relevance of your project. (no more than 1 or 2 paragraphs).
Write your answer here: ____
____
____</td></tr>
<tr><td>5) Describe the purposes and objectives of your project. The purpose of the study is what you are trying to achieve, objectives how you are going to achieve it. Use these examples as a guide:
Script 1:
The purpose of this study is ________________ (If <u>qualitative</u>: understand, describe, develop, discover; If <u>quantitative</u>: measure, establish: the effect, influence, impact, relationship, test the theory) the _____________ (central concept or theory that being studied) in ____________ (unit of analysis or study) through the use of ___________ ____ (methodology).
Script 2:
The purpose of this study is to ______________ (understand, describe, develop, discover, test the theory) the____________ (central concept or theory being studied), which compares _______________ (independent variable) with ____________ (dependent variable) in a group of ______________ (sample) in ______________ (place).</td></tr>
<tr><td>6) Write down some goals (about 2 or 3) for your manuscript.
Write your answer here:
Objective 1: ____
Objective 2: ____
Objective 3: ____</td></tr>
</table>

References

1. Schulz K, Altman D, Moher D, CONSORT Group. CONSORT. 2010 Statement: updated guidelines for reporting parallel group randomised trials. BMC Med. 2010;(8):18. https://doi.org/10.1186/1741-7015-8-18.
2. EQUATOR Network. Enhancing the QUAlity and Transparency Of health Research. Search for reporting guidelines. (2024). https://www.equator-network.org//reporting- guidelines/. Accessed 17 September 2024.
3. Ecarnot F, Seronde MF, Chopard R, Schiele F, Meneveau N. Writing a scientific article: a step-by-step guide for beginners. Eur Geriatr Med. 2015;6:573–379. https://doi.org/10.1016/j.eurger.2015.08.005.
4. Parkar SM, Modi GN, Jani J. Periodontitis as risk factor for acute myocardial infarction: a case control study. Heart Views. 2013;14:5–11. https://doi.org/10.4103/1995-705X.107113.

5. Jacques TS, Sebire NJ. The impact of article titles on citation hits: an analysis of general and specialist medical journals. JRSM Short Rep. 2010;1:2. https://doi.org/10.1258/shorts.2009.100020.
6. Hussain R. Research Topics. Study Guide. School of Health, University of New England. Armidale: UNE. 2003. https://www.une.edu.au/about-une/faculty-of-medicine-and-health/school-of-health/research-in-soh. Accessed 17 September 2024.
7. World Health Organization. Constitution. United Nations. 2024. https://www.who.int/es/about/governance/constitution. Accessed 17 September 2024.
8. The Kipling Society. I Keep Six Honest Serving Men. 2021. https://www.kiplingsociety.co.uk/poem/poems_serving.htm. Accessed 17 September 2024.
9. Cresswell JW. Questions, objectives and hypothesis. In: Qualitative and quantitative approaches. Thousand Oaks: Sage; 1994. p. 69–80. https://psycnet.apa.org/record/1996-97121-000. Accessed 17 September 2024.
10. de Canales FH, Pineda EB. Metodología de la investigación: manual para el desarrollo de personal de salud. Organización Panamericana de la Salud; 1994.
11. Carroll L. A quote from Alice in Wonderland. HTML Edition [electronic resource]. Project Gutenberg. 1997. https://www.gutenberg.org/cache/epub/928/pg928-images.html. Accessed 17 March 2025.
12. Austin Z. How to design and use learning objectives in clinical teaching. The Pharmaceutical Journal, PJ. 2016;296(7885) https://doi.org/10.1211/PJ.2016.20200251.
13. Torre S. Author keywords in PubMed. NLM Tech Bull 2013;(390):e2. https://www.nlm.nih.gov/pubs/techbull/jf13/jf13_pm_keywords.html. Accessed 17 September 2024.

Chapter 7
Preparation of an Original Article: Writing the Materials and Methods Section

Rodrigo Mariño

7.1 Introduction

The objective of the Materials and Methods (M&M) section is to indicate how the study design connects the research question to the results. Starting from a research question, the materials and methods section provides information on how this question will be answered. The content of this section must parallel the presentation of objectives. If there are several secondary objectives, the same order should be followed in the methodology, which will make it easier to read. The answer will be in the results, and therefore no results should be included in this section except for any sections where they must be mentioned to ensure validity or reliability (e.g. kappa of observers, etc.).

This M&M section should provide sufficient information for readers to critically evaluate the methods that will be used. Therefore, we must ensure that the description of the methodology guarantees the obtained results. Generally, this section is written in the past tense: "collected", "asked", etc. when explaining how the results were obtained. The section should provide sufficient details for a reader to replicate the study. This is important, but also a challenge due to word limits.

The level of detail provided will depend on the journal's audience. If it is a dental journal, there is no need to extensively expand upon numerous descriptions that are convention within dental jargon. However, if you are publishing in a non-dental

R. Mariño (✉)
Melbourne Dental School, The University of Melbourne, Melbourne, Australia

Center for Research in Epidemiology, Economics and Oral Public Health (CIEESPO), University de la Frontera, Temuco, Chile

Department of Conservative Dentistry and Oral Health, Riga Stradins University, Riga, Latvia

Monash Health Dental Services, Melbourne, Australia
e-mail: r.marino@unimelb.edu.au

R. Mariño et al. (eds.), *Scientific Writing and Publication Strategies for Oral Health Professionals*, https://doi.org/10.1007/978-3-031-97916-3_7

journal, you may need to add specific details to explain any procedures, indexes, etc. that were used. However, we emphasize that it is not necessary to provide excessive detail, only enough for the reader to understand and replicate the study.

7.2 The Theoretical Framework

The theoretical framework refers to the established theories, concepts, and previous research that form the foundation and guiding principles for a study. It is essential as it provides a solid conceptual foundation for any investigation, placing the study within the context of the existing literature and highlighting the key theories and concepts that guide the analysis. The theoretical framework provides the tools to answer research questions and uses different theories that will explain what we want to study.

In the introduction (see Chap. 6), we talked about the hypotheses to be used. However, in the materials and methods section, these hypotheses are expanded. In the introduction, the hypotheses were mentioned in order to position and give meaning and context to the research question and to the problem to be investigated. More detail on this is provided in the methodology. However, some guidelines for authors may stipulate that the theoretical framework form part of the introduction. This will depend on personal styles or guidelines, but whether it is in the introduction, or in the methodology, you must explain what the theoretical framework of the study is.

7.2.1 What Is a Theory?

A theory is a set of interrelated concepts and the relationships between them, which has a certain level of generalization, can be tested, and which, when tested, acquires validity [1]. They are ideas or concepts, at times abstract, of how the different elements of what you are studying are related. Its function is to provide explanations for aspects of human experience, presenting patterns that do not occur at random [2, 3].

The theoretical framework comes from the review of the literature and will give us knowledge about the existing theory on the topic, its background, the problems and statistical data that will help us identify our variables and the hypotheses that we are going to test. The identification of the theoretical framework is part of our literature review, and it may be an established theory, or a theoretical model that we build ourselves based on our knowledge and experience.

Whilst it is true that clinical studies may differ slightly, there are always theories related to the condition or disease being studied, its underlying biological mechanisms, risk and protective factors, and other relevant variables. The theoretical framework will identify which variables we must collect and how these variables, concepts, or ideas are related in a way that explains the results in the outcome.

A theoretical framework must be specific and have a clear explanation so that the reader can understand why the variables and instruments we are using were chosen, and perhaps even why we analysed the data in a certain way. All this stems from the theoretical framework.

7.3 Materials and Methods Section

The materials and methods section must at a minimum:

- Clearly establish the study design
- Establish the population and sample: size, selection criteria, and the sampling method; that is, how the sample was selected
- Describe, in order, the relevant procedures, laboratory tests, interventions, techniques, analytical methods, etc.
- Define the variables: using operational definitions and measurement levels
- Contain details of the outcome measure(s)/variable(s)
- Describe instruments for measuring variables
- Provide information about the instruments, what are the properties of the instrument that was used (i.e., reliability and validity)
- Discuss ethical considerations
- Provide data analysis methods

In general, in terms of methodology, it is advisable to write your draft in sections, ensuring that each of these points is covered. You can then remove the headers.

7.4 Clearly Establish the Study Design

The M&M section should briefly describe the research design. Remember that a study can use both qualitative or quantitative methodology and design. Most of the studies performed in the health field are quantitative, but in recent years qualitative methodology has been gaining importance.

Explain the study design. If the *methodology is quantitative*: is it cross-sectional, cohort, longitudinal, case–control, is it a controlled clinical trial, community trial, etc.? Figure 7.1 presents the different quantitative study designs [4].

The basic *qualitative research designs* encompass a variety of approaches that seek to understand and interpret human phenomena in depth. There are several commonly used designs for conducting qualitative studies [2]:

- **Phenomenology:** Studies of lived experience.
- **Ethnography:** Issue(s) of interest within a defined culture/subculture.
- **Grounded theory:** Data is collected to develop a theoretical explanation and generate hypothesis for further research.

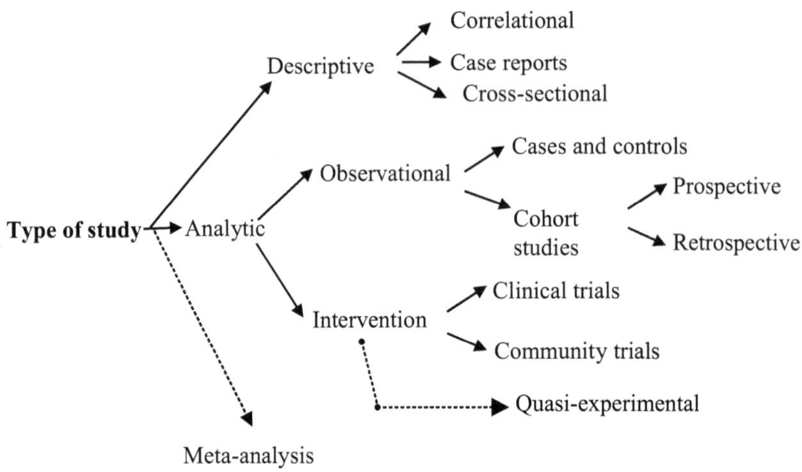

Fig. 7.1 Study design

- **Historic methods:** Examines social phenomena by studying their historical context or their past or past events.
- **Case studies.** Examines a particular case comprehensively and systematically.

7.5 Population and Sample: Size and Sampling Method

The next step is to describe what population is to be studied and how the sample size, selection criteria, or inclusion criteria were determined and to explain what our sampling technique will be, how the sample will be selected and why. That is, justifying the sampling strategy. There are different types of sampling, so we must provide the reader with information as to why one method was selected and not another.

Sampling method is different from sample size. The sample size in quantitative studies depends on several conditions, but certain formulas are used. However, this is independent of how those individuals are going to be selected. This inclusion and exclusion criteria must be defined.

If the goal is to generalize the results to a population, not only is the sample size important, but also how the sample was selected. The number may be correct, but how we select our participants can prevent us from generalizing the results. This sampling method must be described in the methodology. Furthermore, if comparisons are to be made, the statistical power achieved must be indicated to detect differences, if any exist within those groups.

There are different quantitative sampling methods, which can utilise probabilistic methodologies or non-probabilistic methodologies. The use of either probabilistic or non-probabilistic methods does not invalidate the study. The important thing, however, is that it can place limitations on the results of our study, and you must acknowledge these and refer to them in the discussion section. For example, perhaps the sample size calculation indicates that we need 300 participants for our study, but we ended up with only 200. The limitations that a smaller size places upon the study must be discussed. This will be part of the discussion chapter (Chap. 9). As we are still at the methodology stage, having the ideal sample size constitutes perfect planning.

Other times, a study is conceptualized with a probabilistic sample, but in practice, once the data is collected this is no longer possible. What has really happened should be described in the manuscript. There are several situations in which probabilistic studies cannot be done.

As mentioned before, the use of smaller samples or non-probability sampling does not necessarily invalidate a result. There are certain situations that, due to the characteristics of the population we are going to study, can only be studied through non-probabilistic sampling. For example, in many cases there are no lists of all potential participants for a given study, which would enable the use of probabilistic methods. This is important and must be kept in mind as we will have to refer to any sampling methods we use and their limitations in the discussion.

Qualitative methods generally use small, highly selective samples, because the goal is to obtain those that are rich in information. Therefore, they will always use non-probabilistic methods where informants are selected based on what we want to study and the individuals that we want to identify. In qualitative studies, the size of the sample is not defined in the research protocol because we seek to identify individuals that are "rich in information", which is why qualitative studies usually use convenience or purposeful sampling. The number of participants then increases until a so-called "saturation" of information occurs. That is, a point is reached where no further new information or ideas arise, and the collection of ideas appears to be complete.

Describe, in a chronological sequence, procedures, laboratory tests, interventions, techniques, analytical methods, etc.

Once the study design, population, and sample are established, we must describe the data collection procedures. This must be done in a chronological manner. Describe when we started, how it started, how it ended, what procedures were followed.

Describe, in detail and in an orderly manner, how the data from the study unit was obtained. Indicate what procedures were used to ensure the quality of the data. Indicate whether this data already existed, for example if it is secondary data, or whether you collected it yourself. One example of secondary data is when we take it from clinical records or health records.

7.6 Variables: Operational Definitions and Measurement Level

The methodology identifies and clearly defines the variables to be used and how they are going to be measured. Variables can be measured with different scales. For example, age is a variable that may seem very clear to us, but we must describe how it was defined for our study, and with which scale it will be measured. The age variable can be defined in terms of number of years, but I can also define age in groups, from 5 to 10 years, from 11 to 15 years, etc. In this case, it is no longer a continuous variable, but rather an ordinal one. I can also measure age as "Over 35 years old" or "35 less years old", which is a categorical variable.

The scale to be used comes from the theory and what the literature tells us. If we are going to use years, or months, or even days, it should be because the literature tells us that this variable is important, and that it must be measured in a certain way. It is too late if after we collect data, we realize that instead of collecting age as over or under 35, a little more detail was needed. This is why scale is important and forms part of the foundation of the study.

Income can also be described and measured in different ways. We must describe in the methodology whether income refers to monthly income, income after deducting taxes, or before. Whatever you use, it must be defined in the methodology.

Some variables must be operationalized since they do not exist as such. The methodology must also briefly describe this.

It is also important that when data is collected, for example using a self-completed form, that the instructions and questions to be asked are clear for the participants. For example, indicate the units used, whether it be kilos, grams, milligrams, minutes, seconds, etc. As mentioned, if the question asked is about income, participants may respond in different ways unless the instructions are clearly stated. Any inconsistency in the responses may render the information incomparable, or unusable. Therefore, this must be defined and clarified in the methodology.

The theoretical framework and the literature review will define which are the dependent and independent variables. The theoretical framework should also describe why these variables, and not others, will be used to answer the research question. Of course, there may be situations where this is considered obvious and you do not have to give too much detail, but in other circumstances it might not be as clear. For example, why was sex used? Why was age used? Why was education or income level used, etc.?

7.7 Instruments for Data Collection

The M&M must indicate and describe the type of instrument used and provide a justification for that selection. To give an example, in recent years there has been a tendency to use the quality-of-life variable in relation to oral health. There are several quality-of-life instruments related to oral health available [5]. Perhaps the most used is the Oral Health Impact Profile (OHIP) [6], but there are others. We must provide a justification as to why we selected a particular quality-of-life instrument, among all those instruments that can potentially be used, and justify why we are using that one and not another.

If an existing instrument is going to be used, its reliability and validity must be described. There are several ways to establish the validity of an instrument. Currently, most journals will request this information. If this is unknown, indicate how they were specifically evaluated in that study. If you are going to use a new instrument, you must explain the steps that were followed to construct that instrument and provide information on how reliability and validity were measured. If other researchers validated it, explain how they did it and provide the corresponding references. This evaluation must be done before beginning data collection. If you do it after data collection and realize that the instrument is not valid or unreliable, it is too late.

The methodology must also provide information on any training or calibration of examiners. If a calibration exercise was conducted, include the results. It is not necessary to describe the whole process, but to indicate that the interviewers were trained for data collection, that the examiners were trained and calibrated, for example specifically in the measurement of dental caries, and add the results of this calibration.

If pilot studies were conducted, explain and describe how they were done, and whether the results of that pilot changed the original methodology. For example, whether the instrument was changed, whether the study design was changed, whether the data collection methodology was adjusted, etc. If there were no changes, also indicate this so that the reader has the information.

There are many ways to collect *qualitative data*. However, in general, the researcher is the real instrument [7]. This is because the quality, type, and quantity of data largely depend on the skills of the researcher [8]. Qualitative researchers follow a series of techniques to collect data: a questionnaire, generally with open questions, an interview, focus groups, diaries, etc. However, other methods are concurrently employed. For example, observation. From a qualitative point, any gestures, for example, that a participant makes may be very important. For this purpose, field notes and videos are relevant and must also be described in the methods section.

The concepts of validity and reliability also apply to qualitative research [2]. Reliability refers to whether the records or transcripts are consistent with what occurred [2]. The audios or videos of the interviews, for example, or focus groups, are reviewed to confirm that the transcription accurately reflects what happened in the interview or focus group, and this is achieved by reviewing the videos or audios.

The validity of the information refers to whether the explanation that comes from what the data describes or corresponds to what really happened during data collection. If using qualitative methods, this work is done by coding the texts. Therefore, the coding that a researcher puts in must be validated by another member of the team. Interview coding, for example, is usually repeated, and we verify whether different researchers can attain the same coding. This information must be included in the M&M of a qualitative manuscript.

7.8 Ethical Considerations

Ethical considerations must also be included in the M&M. It is not necessary to expand on all ethical issues, but to minimally indicate by which ethics committee or ethics committees the study was approved, as it might have been more than one, and provide the registration number. In fact, this number is now requested as part of the process of submitting manuscripts for review. Refer to the author guidelines and what they ask for.

7.9 Data Analysis

This section does not report the results of the analyses but indicates how the data was manipulated and analysed to draw conclusions. The section should relate the analysis that was done back to the objectives. You can even structure this subsection in those exact terms; *to answer objective 1 or research question 1, the researchers will use this test and analytical procedures. For objective 2, we will use this test and analytical procedure*, etc. However, this must be posed in relation to the specific objectives. Do not use generic descriptions, but rather specify which analysis was done to answer the research question. In fact, the entire M&M section must relate back to the objectives of the study or research questions.

7.9.1 Quantitative Data Analysis

If a *quantitative methodology* is used, a statistical analysis section must include descriptive statistics, where only the variables are described. This can be done through inferential statistics in which parametric or non-parametric methods are used.

Indicate the preset *p*-value. In the planning stage, we decide what our level of statistical significance will be. Keep in mind that a *p*-value is just a probability of something happening. A value of 0.05, or 0.01, or 0.001, does not indicate that one variable has more effect than another, but only the probability that something happens by chance. If that probability is low, it can be concluded that something influenced the results, and this factor is our intervention or experiment.

As part of this subsection, you may need to describe how the assumptions behind the parametric tests (i.e., normality, homogeneity of variance, and independence of observations) were verified. We are not going to go into detail on this, but at a minimum, it should be confirmed that the assumptions under parametric tests were checked. It is not necessary to go in detail about how this was done, or the results. However, it is possible that a reviewer or examiner may request that the details of this information be included.

If multivariate methods are used, there are other important practical issues to review. Multivariate methods, such as logistic regression and linear regression, are based on a straight line. Therefore, the data must be linear. If not, the results from that type of analysis may not be valid. For example, if we have a U-shaped effect, or a V-shaped effect, or an inverted V-shaped effect, or an inverted U-shaped effect, it is very powerful but may not manifest using linear regression because the shape itself is not linear. The absence of multicollinearity should also be checked. That is, the variables are not highly correlated. For example, education and income are closely related. If the two variables were placed in a multivariate model, this could cause issues such as unstable coefficient estimates or decreased interpretability. It must also be demonstrated that there were no outliers, as these are extreme values that will change our results.

At a minimum, in one sentence, and without too much detail, you should indicate that these assumptions were examined.

7.9.2 *Qualitative Data Analysis*

Qualitative data cannot be analysed using statistical methods. This data does not consist of numbers, but rather texts, or silences, or gestures, etc. This is all valuable information for a qualitative study. For this type of analysis, the first thing qualitative researchers do is immerse themselves into the data. This is done by reading and rereading the transcriptions, the field notes, watching and rewatching videos that indicate where the informant, for example, blushed, or changed posture, or showed discomfort.

Once the investigator has been "immersed" into the data, inductive methods are used to make sense of the information and to extract and synthesize its meaning [1]. The analysis is done using the summary and interpretation of the findings, usually in narrative form, which can become very complicated if done manually and may take a long time. There are computer programs, for example, NVivo (https://lumivero.com/products/nvivo-qualitative-data-analysis-software/) and Atlas.ti (https://atlasti.com/), that facilitate this qualitative analysis. In addition, this software allows us to identify agreements between coders. This will also help them demonstrate the validity of the information.

7.10 Final Remarks

It was mentioned that the M&M section might be the shortest section of a manuscript, but a balance must be achieved between providing detail and the essential elements required. Always ask yourself, could a reader repeat the methods used in the study? The methodology must provide sufficient information so that the study can be replicated. See Box 7.1, which presents a summary of points to remember when writing the materials and methods section.

You can use subheadings for these separate subsections when writing the M&M and then delete them but ensure you have included all components. In M&M, there is no need to comment on the methods mentioned and, above all, do not include results. Follow the guidelines and instructions of the journal.

Remember the five Rs that must be included in the methodology [9]. The methodology has to be relevant, including only the information which pertains to the study. It must be rigorous in its description of what was done. It must be concise, in the sense of words chosen. It should indicate what resources were necessary to obtain information in terms of questionnaires, type of statistical software, etc. In addition, they must be replicable [7].

Box 7.1 Points to Remember When Writing the Materials and Methods Section
Methodology Points to remember

- Do not comment on methods
- Reference already published methods; a summary may be appropriate.
- See instructions on how to cite patented products (e.g., dental materials); in parentheses? footnote? endnote?
- Paragraphs; use of subheadings?
- Flowcharts if there are multiple groups/treatments? Abbreviated quantitative units
- Length of the section.
- Follow any equator guideline: https://www.equator-network.org/reporting-guidelines/
- **Can readers repeat the methods?**

5 Rs: Relevant; Rigorous; Rapid; Required resources; Repeatable

In summary, at a minimum, the methodology should include:

- **Sample**: describe who was included (and who was not), how many, why the sampling strategy was used, and how the sample will be selected.
- **Data collection**: indicate (a) the instruments and (b) the procedures. If an existing instrument is to be used, it must be described, and its psychometric properties (validity and reliability) indicated. If an instrument is to be built, outline the steps to follow, the pilot test, preliminary data, etc.
- **Procedures**: indicate how the data will be collected and what procedures are used to ensure its quality.
- **Data analysis**: indicate procedures and statistical packages, but not the results of these tests.

A researcher will never have absolute control of what happens in a study. There can always be errors, which are impossible to avoid entirely. However, an error could be random, or it could be systematic bias. In the methodology, it is necessary to indicate how this error was handled, or demonstrate to the reader, the reviewer, the examiner, that this possibility was reduced to an absolute minimum. In addition, keep in mind that any study will have limitations, and we must be open and transparent about the limitations of our study design and methodology. They are not necessarily going to invalidate a study, but you must tell the reader, or the reviewer, or the examiner that you are aware of any limitations that this may have imposed on the study. This will be discussed in Chap. 9.

Given that reading the materials is only one aspect of the learning process, the chapter includes an Appendix (Activity 7.1) to facilitate the immediate application of new concepts and knowledge.

Appendix

Activity 7.1
1) Identify the theoretical elements necessary to support the study (2 or 3 paragraphs). Write your answer here: _
2) Make a list of all the variables you used in your study. Write your answer here: Is an operational definition of any of the variables you use needed? If necessary, write thedefinition(s) here: _
3) Select the main variables required to answer the research question Write your answer here: _
4) Outline the relationships between the variables and identify the relationship betweenthe variables and the hypotheses (if your study is descriptive, develop the implicit hypotheses) (1 or 2 paragraphs). Write your answer here: _
5) Indicate the sampling strategy you used in your study (1 or 2 paragraphs). **a. Include a justification for that strategy.** **b. Indicate what size sample you think you will need** **i.** Justify your sample size and describe your calculation. Write your answer here: _
6) Indicate which data collection strategy you used in your study (procedures andinstruments) (2 or 3 paragraphs). Write your answer here: _

(continued)

(continued)

7) Indicate what data analysis strategy you used in your study (1 or 2 paragraphs). Write your answer here: _
8) Discuss ethical issues. Informed consent, use of underage, etc. If you have it, includethe ethics approval number (1 or 2 sentences). Write your answer here: _

References

1. Blaikie N. Designing social research: the logic of anticipation. 2nd ed. Oxford: Polity; 2009.
2. Borbasi S, Langford R, Jackson D. Navigating the maze of nursing research: an interactive learning adventure. Sydney: Elsevier Australia; 2003.
3. Wingood G, Di Clemente R. The use of psychosocial models for guiding the design and implementation of HIV prevention interventions. In: Gibney L, Di Clemente R, Vermund S, editors. Preventing HIV in developing countries. Boston: Springer; 2002. p. 187–204. https://link.springer.com/chapter/10.1007/0-306-47157-4_9. Accessed 18 Nov 2024.
4. Hennekens C, Buring J. Epidemiology in medicine. Boston: Little, Brown. Scientific Research Publishing; 1987.
5. McGrath C, Rogers SN. Overview of instruments used to assess quality of lifein dentistry. In: Preedy VR, Watson RR, editors. Handbook of disease burdens and quality of life measures. New York: Springer; 2010. p. 145–59. https://doi.org/10.1007/978-0-387-78665-0_8.
6. Slade G, Spencer A. Development and evaluation of the Oral Health Impact Profile. Community Dent Health. 1994;11:3–11. PMID: 8193981
7. Pezalla A, Pettigrew J, Miller-Day M. Researching the researcher-as-instrument: an exercise in interviewer self-reflexivity. Qual Res. 2012;12:165–85. https://doi.org/10.1177/1487941111422107.
8. Burns N, Grove S. Investigación en enfermería. 3rd ed. Madrid: Elsevier; 2009.
9. Peek C, Glasgow R, Stange K, Klesges L, Purcell E, Kessler R. The 5 R's: an emerging bold standard for conducting relevant research in a changing world. Ann Fam Med. 2014;12:447–55. https://doi.org/10.1370/afm.1688.

Chapter 8
Preparation of an Original Article: Writing the Results Section

Rodrigo Mariño and Maura Klenner

8.1 Introduction

Many researchers would like to include the analysis of all the variables that were collected in the study in this section, but this challenge proves more than impossible when there is limited space or time to do so. The alternative is to only include those that will be used in the analysis. For example, if you are going to test the distribution of caries according to age and sex, you must include descriptive information about these ages and sexes at the beginning of the results section. Then describe the main variables, for example, the caries history index (DMF index), its mean, standard deviation, range, etc., or frequency of visits to the dentist, each described individually.

In the results section the rule is to first show the forest, and then the trees [1]. That is, begin generally then become more specific. If there is a sample, describe the sample, by age, sex, education, etc. For example, begin with a description of how many participants there were, how many trials were done, etc. and indicate what the response rate was. This information is important, because it tells the reader the external validity or generalizability of the results.

R. Mariño (✉)
Melbourne Dental School, The University of Melbourne, Melbourne, Australia

Center for Research in Epidemiology, Economics and Oral Public Health (CIEESPO), University de la Frontera, Temuco, Chile

Department of Conservative Dentistry and Oral Health, Riga Stradins University, Riga, Latvia

Monash Health Dental Services, Melbourne, Australia
e-mail: r.marino@unimelb.edu.au

M. Klenner
Departamento de Lenguas, Literatura y Comunicaciȯn, University de la Frontera, Temuco, Chile
e-mail: maura.klenner@ufrontera.cl

R. Mariño et al. (eds.), *Scientific Writing and Publication Strategies for Oral Health Professionals*, https://doi.org/10.1007/978-3-031-97916-3_8

As its name indicates, this section presents the results or the findings of a study. Although it seems obvious, it is not unusual to find an aspect of the methodology in the discussion in some manuscripts. To clarify, methodology should always go in the material and methods section and the interpretation or analysis of the results in the discussion section.

Of course, it is always possible as part of the introduction of a new paragraph, to remind the reader or examiner what the hypotheses, research questions, or the methodology used are, that is, it is indicating that this or that test was carried out and that these are the results. However, if this is done, it should be brief and only as a reminder of what is being presented.

8.2 Practical Issues

The results section is generally written in the past tense: "it was collected", "it was measured", etc. and does not use references as they are our own results. Only the results that were included in this section will be part of the discussion and will go in the abstract. The abstract, and much less the discussion, cannot present data that was not described in the results section. Also, you must always be honest and transparent with what was done. Present the results, and then in the discussion you can let the reader make a judgement about their validity.

Keep in mind that the discussion section discusses or comments on the results. Therefore, in the results section avoid using phrases like: "Without a doubt…"; "Surprisingly…", or similar, as this indicates a discussion of the results.

The results of a calibration are not results of the study but part of the methodology, where you demonstrate that the examiner, or an instrument, was calibrated and trained to make the assessments and measurements, although they are a form of result, they are not part of the results section as such, but part of the methodology. Likewise, providing information about how the assumptions that support the parametric tests were evaluated, for example that the distribution is normal, is part of the methodology and not the research question.

By convention, when a sentence begins with a number, it should be phrased as words and not digits (e.g., "Seven hundred and fifty participants", not "750 participants"). There is also, by convention, a rule that when the numbers are smaller than 10, for example "6", they are written in words. From 10 onwards numbers are written in figures, but text will always be used to begin a sentence. However, these are only conventions, and they can also vary from one journal to another. This is why it is important to review the author's guidelines.

Generally, in a quantitative article, the results section is the shortest section but also the most important. Therefore, we must always identify which data we will present and how we are going to present it. If you exceed the limits, not so much of words but of pages, some journals will charge per extra page. This amount may be a little less for online publications, but we must always be rigorous and avoid including what is not absolutely necessary, always following the word limit indications.

In cases where the results section might get very complex, it is important to establish a clear structure at the beginning. That is, indicate in the first paragraph of the section how the different aspects of the results will be presented and organized. This strategy helps to orient the reader and facilitates understanding of the information presented in this section.

Ideally, present your results following the same order in which the objectives of the study were stated. Also, follow the order of result presentation if including tables, graphs, etc.

To improve the flow of the text, make a transition between different divisions or paragraphs of the results. For example, at the end of a paragraph, introduce the next one to avoid independent paragraphs.

If you are going to compare two or more groups, describe whether those groups were the same or different at the beginning. This is because if we are going to test a technique, the groups must be equal or equivalent at the beginning to demonstrate that the effect is due to the intervention. That is part of the presentation of results. However, consider that it is also possible that the hypothesis might actually require that the groups be different to begin with.

If data has been manipulated, deleted, or combined in any way, indicate this where appropriate. For example, if we are working with dental caries history, we present our data and say that "only those who were dentate were included in the analysis presented below", or "edentulous participants are not part of the analysis that follows". Also include if any variable categories were combined. Of course, when this data manipulation is part of the final results it is then part of the methodology, but it should be repeated in the relevant section if it relates to a particular aspect of the results.

A balance must be achieved between describing each result and including only those that are significant. Remember that you cannot put all the information in a single manuscript. Tables and graphs are used to highlight data that is important, not to present all the information. There is a limitation on the number of tables, usually two or three, and the guidelines for authors specify this limit.

When using tables, begin with a description in the text: "Table 1 shows that…" and guide the reader through the text. For example, "In column 2 of Table 1", or "In the third line of Table 1", etc. Guide the reader to find the information you are referring to.

Then, add the statistical results that support those results. Some formats only ask to indicate the *p*-value (e.g. 0.05 or 0.01), while other formats request all the information. For example, for an ANOVA test: [F (3,58) = 5.79, $p < 0.05$]. Likewise, verify if the exact *p*-values must be formatted exactly as they were obtained from a statistical program (e.g. $p = 0.026$), or as less than a certain level of statistical significance (i.e., <0.05; <0.01, etc.). However, it is important to standardize the style to be used throughout the manuscript. This is outlined in the guidelines to authors. Follow the instructions and if there are none, be consistent and use a single format. These are not particularly important for the findings being presented, but they are distracting for the reader, or the reviewer, or the examiner, which is why consistency is so important.

Regarding the *p*-values, please keep in mind that they do not necessarily provide evidence that a null hypothesis is right or wrong. It might be that the sample size is very small and therefore there is not enough statistical power to detect any differences that exist. On the other hand, a statistically significant *p*-value may be the result of differences that are not clinically significant. It may also happen when the sample size is too large, as even very small differences will be significant. Therefore, always evaluate and be critical of the results you obtained.

We must also remember that a p-value of "0.00" is not theoretically possible. The statistical packages will round off and set zero, but in theory, the curve never crosses the x-axis. Therefore, theoretically there will never be a value of $p = 0.00$. This is why it is important to correctly interpret the value provided by the statistical packages. The probability may be 0.00001, or smaller, but there must be a "1" somewhere. Again, while that does necessarily change the result, it will distract the reader or the reviewer.

Also, keep in mind that when reporting statistical results, it is important to emphasize that p-values indicate statistical significance but do not provide any information on the magnitude of that difference. The 95% confidence intervals (CIs) give a clearer understanding of the magnitude and precision of the effect or difference, helping us understand the practical impact of the treatments.

For non-statistically significant results, it is not necessary to enter the specific p-values of the result but only to indicate that, for example, sex or level of education was not significant for a history of dental caries, because of limitations placed by word count. However, a non-significant difference can be as important as a significant difference. Therefore, this information must be indicated even if the difference was not statistically significant. Of course, this will depend on the research questions and what is being presented.

8.3 How to Present Data

Data can be presented or described pictorially, for example in tables, graphs, or figures, or be described numerically in text as proportions, frequencies, measures of central tendency and measures of dispersion, etc. Always remember not to go beyond what is necessary to describe your findings. To save words, you can avoid presenting the obvious. For example, 51% of the participants were male and 49% were female—one is the complement of the other. It may not be necessary to explicitly state it.

8.3.1 Some Considerations of Tables and Graphs

If you are going to use tables, graphs, charts, or figures to describe the data, do not repeat the same information in the text and in graphic form. A graph, a table, etc. serves to highlight the most important or relevant findings. Decide how best to present your results. This will depend on personal preference, guidelines to authors, and how the data can be made easier to understand or follow.

- Tables, graphs, figures must be independent and self-explanatory. Therefore, the reader should be able to understand their content without having to resort to other sources of clarification, for example the results section.

- Titles should be clear and answer the questions: who?, how?, where?, and when? The title can be placed above the table or below. This is up to personal preference unless defined in the guidelines.
- Codes, abbreviations, or symbols must be explained in detail in the footnotes at the bottom of the table, figure, or graph.
- Of course, there is no need to explain matters that are obvious, but there are situations where abbreviations vary from profession to profession and therefore it is necessary to define them, especially when they published in non-dental journals, for example.
- Make sure that all tables, graphs, figures, etc., are presented in numerical order. Ensure that there are no errors in the format, and that there is consistency in the fonts and their sizes as requested by the journal.

When tables are used:

- Rows and columns should have clear and concise titles.
- If units of measurement are used, indicate them. If they use abbreviations such as mg for milligrams, state that "mg" means milligrams.
- Indicate the totals of the columns and rows, if they include numerical data. Make sure that the percentages add up to 100%, not 100.1% or 99.9%, as statistical packages can sometimes round off.
- If the figures do not match because of missing values, it should be indicated at the bottom of the table that it is possible that the values may not add up because of this. For example, if we have 150 participants but the results indicate that 50 are male and 99 are female, this is because one participant did not include the information. Therefore, at the bottom of the table the numbers may not add up due to missing values.
- Do not include more information than a typical reader can interpret easily. Do not try to summarize all our information on a single table.

A graph is another way to represent information using a coordinate system. In addition to what was outlined above:

- Do not place more lines or symbols than the eye can easily see and understand.
- If more than one variable is shown, label them clearly. Be careful with the colours. Whether in black and white or in colours, make sure it is easy to differentiate the variables within the graph.
- Remember that graphs use the coordinate axis, therefore, each axis has units clearly indicated.
- The separation between intervals must be equal, if they are equal intervals. Scale breaks can be used in certain situations, but this must be clearly identified.
- Use the correct graph. For example, if values are not continuous, a histogram cannot be used.

Follow the guidelines regarding requirements for where to place tables and figures or graphs. In some situations, the guidelines request for them to be included in the manuscript and other times as a separate file. Other times, the title must be placed separately from the table and so on.

It may be that the journal will use the table, graph, or figure, exactly as they are submitted. Make sure from the beginning that the requirements are being followed, and the quality of the graphics, tables, and figures is in the requested file format. There are many that can be used, such as JPEG, PNG, GIF, etc. You should also pay attention to the size or resolution of the indicated pixels. For example, a graph provided in PDF format will not have the necessary quality. Follow the instructions, because it will only be returned to you for improvement, or worse, be published exactly as it was sent, even if it is of poor quality.

8.3.2 Multivariate Analysis

Most of the time, a bivariate analysis will not be sufficient to support your conclusion. Multivariate analysis allows for a more complete understanding and allows stronger conclusions to be drawn based on the relationships observed. A multivariate analysis can be very important when drawing the conclusions of the study. Without performing this analysis, there is a risk of drawing conclusions that are incomplete or incorrect. Without this analysis, individual effects of each independent variable and their influence cannot be determined without taking the effects of other variables into account.

8.4 Qualitative Data

Most of this chapter concerns how to present quantitative data using statistics, but there are also qualitative results. The qualitative results section is a little different. In general, qualitative data is presented with titles or subtitles according to themes or categories which have been identified in the analysis.

Unlike a quantitative manuscript, in a qualitative one the results section is the longest. In a qualitative manuscript the discussion and presentation of data can be done at the same time and a mix of the two is allowed, unlike in a quantitative manuscript where there is a clear separation and structure between results discussion. Furthermore, qualitative manuscripts tend to be longer than quantitative ones, because the data itself is text and will therefore take up more words.

Qualitative studies do not use statistical tests. They may present a numerical description of the participants, for example, their average age or sex distribution, but the objective of qualitative methodology is to generate hypotheses and not test them. The bulk of the result is the textual analysis of the information that was collected.

Qualitative samples are smaller. A sample of 15, 20, or even less, is acceptable whereas a sample of 15 or 20 in quantitative data is considered to be very small. This is because in qualitative research the objective may be to present or describe atypical cases. In quantitative research, an extreme value (i.e., an outlier) may affect the average but in qualitative methodology, but this participant is important because they deviate and therefore may suggest a topic in need of exploration. The objective is to explore why the participant is an outlier [2].

Nowadays there is more fluidity in quantitative journals, and they also accept qualitative manuscripts. If the reviewer is from a quantitative background, they may not evaluate it any differently because the sample is very small or not representative, for example. In a qualitative manuscript the aim is different.

8.5 Final Remarks

In a quantitative manuscript, we must be selective with the information that we are going to present. The results section is not about throwing data at the reader, because they will not remember it [1]. Therefore, we cannot include everything and must focus only on what answers our main research question or questions [3]. This is not just due to space and text limitations—the intention is for them to remember finding that is being presented.

In this section, you must only describe the results. The discussion section will examine their implications or explain why they were obtained. The reader or examiner should be able to understand the data and its implications before even moving on to this section [3]. That is, when reading the data, they should already be thinking about what the possible implications or discussion of the results are.

Once again, consider the use of paragraphs and subheadings to facilitate flow. Readers will appreciate fluidity in the presentation of the data. The results section should emphasize what is important and make it easier for the reader to find the answer to the research question we have proposed.

Do not present data that will not be discussed. If a piece of data is not discussed, it should not be in the results, unless it is background information for an analysis that is going to be done. On the other hand, do not ignore those results that do not support the conclusions. This could be important, as it might provide another perspective on those results, or apply to a different population. For example, the current cohorts of older adults are different from 20 years ago. As such, current results may not generate the same results we had previously, creating a conflict. Therefore, we must let the data tell us the story rather than forcing a conclusion.

Review examples of results sections or sample documents that a journal has previously included, or not included, look at the journals where you want to publish your data, and see how the results section is structured and what are the conventions are for the content, extension, and visualization of data [3].

As stated previously, writing a manuscript is an iterative process, going through several cycles until the results section is finished or the manuscript is finalized and can be submitted for peer review. As an iterative process, teamwork is essential and there is very rarely a single author. This is why it is important to collaborate with your co-authors and consider their contributions in the writing process.

If you are out to describe the truth, leave elegance to the tailor.—Albert Einstein

Regarding the presentation of data, we must remember Einstein's quote that highlights the importance of describing the truth with simplicity. Rather than focusing on attracting the greatest number of people, we must communicate clearly and simply, prioritizing those who are interested in our research.

The chapter also incorporates an Appendix (Activity 8.1), which is designed to facilitate the practical application of concepts and knowledge, as described in the chapter.

Appendix

Activity 8.1
1) Describe how many people participated and indicate the response rate. Describe the sample (age, sex, education, etc.) and other socioeconomic variables. **Describe other key variables. For example, use of oral health services; DMFT, periodontal health, etc.** **Write your response: ____________________** ____________________ ____________________
2) Describe other analyses that were conducted. For example, comparisons of initial values for main outcome variables. **Write your response: ____________________** ____________________ ____________________
3) Describe the results of the analysis used to test the hypothesis on the main outcome variable/Your specific research question. **If there is more than one research question, describe the results of all.** **Write your response:** **Research Question 1: ____________________** ____________________ **Research Question 2: ____________________** ____________________ **Research Question 3: ____________________** **4) Describe other analysis you performed. For example, multivariate analysis.** **Write your answer here: ____________________** ____________________ **5) Provide a list and layouts for the tables and figures you want to include in your research paper. Please note that most journals have limits on the number of tables and figures you can include in your manuscript, so you should only show the essential tables and figures (maximum 3 tables/graphs in total).** **Write your answer here: ____________________** ____________________ ____________________

(*continued*)

(continued)

6) Checklist:	
a. You have completed data collection and analyzed the results.	**Yes No**
a. You have included all the results that are relevant to my research questions.	**Yes No**
b. You have concisely and objectively reported each result, including relevant descriptive statistics and inferential statistics.	**Yes No**
c. You have described whether each hypothesis was supported or refuted.	**Yes No**
d. Have you used tables and figures to illustrate my results when appropriate.	**Yes No**
e. All tables and figures are correctly labelled and referenced in the text.	**Yes No**
f. Have you not provided subjective interpretation or speculation about the meaning of the results.	**Yes No**

References

1. Bem DJ. Writing the empirical journal article. In: Darley JM, Zanna MP, Roediger HL, editors. The compleat academic: A career guide. 2nd ed. Washington, DC: American Psychological Association; 2004. p. 185–219.
2. Greenland S, Senn SJ, Rothman KJ, Carlin JB, Poole C, Goodman SN, Altman DG. Statistical tests, P values, confidence intervals, and power: a guide to misinterpretations. Eur J Epidemiol. 2016;31:337–50. https://doi.org/10.1007/s10654-016-0149-3.
3. Anderson C. Presenting and evaluating qualitative research. Am J Pharm Educ. 2010;74:141. https://doi.org/10.5688/aj7408141.
4. Snyder N, Foltz C, Lendner M, Vaccaro AR. How to write an effective results section. Clin Spine Surg. 2019;32:295–6. https://doi.org/10.1097/BSD.0000000000000845.

Chapter 9
Preparation of an Original Article: Writing the Discussion Section

Rodrigo Mariño and Estefanía Patiño-Ramon

9.1 Introduction

In Chaps. 2 and 6 it was mentioned that in a research project there are several questions to answer, but the main one would be the significance, the "So what?". This answer is provided in the discussion section. This is where the authors talk about the "So what?", discussing the consequences and importance of the findings obtained from the research while emphasizing what is new and novel about the study, so that it is not just another publication.

As researchers, we aspire to have an impact, and that impact is shown in the citations of our publications. Therefore, although a publication is in itself an achievement, the true success lies in the impact, specifically, the number of times it is cited by other researchers. That is, how the information and discoveries made have been used by other researchers. Of course, a recent publication will not have that many citations but over the years, the impact of the publication should become apparent. In Chap. 3 a series of indices measuring this impact were presented.

The previous chapter noted that the most important part of a manuscript is the results section, which provides the presentation and analysis of the data of a study.

R. Mariño (✉)
Melbourne Dental School, The University of Melbourne, Melbourne, Australia

Center for Research in Epidemiology, Economics and Oral Public Health (CIEESPO), University de la Frontera, Temuco, Chile

Department of Conservative Dentistry and Oral Health, Riga Stradins University, Riga, Latvia

Monash Health Dental Services, Melbourne, Australia
e-mail: r.marino@unimelb.edu.au

E. Patiño-Ramon
Universidad Católica de Cuenca, Cuenca, Ecuador
e-mail: erika.patino@est.ucacue.edu.ec

R. Mariño et al. (eds.), *Scientific Writing and Publication Strategies for Oral Health Professionals*, https://doi.org/10.1007/978-3-031-97916-3_9

However, the discussion section is equally important because it puts those results into perspective. The discussion is the creative aspect of the study and publication, where the authors utilize their critical and analytical abilities to synthesize ideas and information, contextualizing the results within the existing literature on a topic.

The purpose is to describe, interpret, and emphasize the importance of the findings considering the existing knowledge on the topic under study. The goal is to build on known information and create new knowledge, which must be explained and analysed in light of the findings of the study. The discussion should connect the initial literature review, research questions, and hypotheses to the findings. However, it is not just about merely repeating the findings but rather connecting what was known at the beginning with the new knowledge obtained, which is where the creative aspect lies.

The discussion should clarify how the study advanced our understanding of a problem. The current state of knowledge was previously presented in the introduction section, while the research generates new knowledge, as detailed in the results section. The discussion contextualizes that new knowledge critically, in context with what was already known. This section should answer the question: What does this study add?

Additionally, as mentioned in Chap. 2, research is a cycle in which new knowledge is created, continually generating new questions as it evolves. Therefore, a good analysis and discussion should provide guidelines on how to continue this line of research. The discussion must also address a second question: What are the next steps to follow in this line of research? It should encompass not only new questions, but also how to collect and analyse the information moving forward.

This section should demonstrate the researchers' capacity to think critically about the topic, develop creative solutions based on the findings, and formulate a deeper understanding of the problem being studied. The discussion explores the meaning of the study, its implications for other areas of research and professional practice, and how our research can improve situations and enhance practice as it relates to the "So what?", "What is this for?" questions.

The discussion is not meant to be a simple descriptive report of the results. It must include elements of creativity and innovative thinking. However, any interpretation offered must be founded on evidence. This presents a paradox: how can we offer creative insights while relaying on what we already know? Nonetheless, it is about forging new connections that may not be immediately apparent and generating new hypotheses and research questions. Thus, the creative element extends beyond a simple description of the results.

Albert Einstein once said: "*Imagination is more important than knowledge*". That means we must employ creative thinking, but that creativity must be grounded on evidence and a logical framework.

9.2 The Content

The discussion section begins by highlighting the importance of the study and its contribution to addressing the existing gaps in a specific line of research, as well as indicating the new and innovative knowledge obtained through the study. If applicable, it should mention how the results filled knowledge gaps that were previously overlooked or inadequately described in the literature.

Next, the discussion should address whether the results align with the explanation for the observed outcomes. It is important not to limit a study to whether the results were statistically significant or not. Often there is a bias towards only publishing only statistically significant findings, however, non-significant results can offer valuable insights just as significant results do (Organizing Academic Research Papers).

Recently, a colleague and I submitted a manuscript for peer review that presented a study with no statistically significant findings. My colleague questioned the value of publishing it; however, the manuscript indicated that these results contributed to our understanding of the specific situation studied, detailing the population and its sociodemographic context. Thus, even without significant outcomes, there was a notable contribution to knowledge. It is for the peer review to decide whether this contribution was indeed significant. The manuscript also explained why our results diverged from the existing literature, thereby linking our findings to the body of existing knowledge on the topic.

Therefore, if the results differ from what was expected according to existing literature, it is essential to provide explanations for these discrepancies based on available evidence. It is crucial to highlight any unusual or unforeseen trends in the results. A vital aspect of research is not only providing answers but also generating new questions that require further investigation. Emphasizing these new inquiries, along with an acknowledgment that the current study's design may not have addressed them, suggests how future studies with different designs could explore these issues.

Additionally, it is important to contextualize our findings within the broader research landscape. This requires more than merely stating that our study is "similar to a study in..." or that the effect was greater or lower than another study's findings. Instead, the discussion should explain how the results can be generally applied. Therefore, any references to other research must be relevant, as not all studies can meaningfully be compared to each other.

The discussion section must engage with the existing body of evidence and consider what other researchers have discovered, placing our results in that context. The goal is not only to describe past research but to critically connect our results to the wider literature. While a literature review was included in the introduction of the study, an additional review in the discussion may incorporate both the references used initially and new ones that relate to the comparisons being drawn. This section should therefore feature a discussion and analysis of what has been previously established by other researchers, further situating our findings within that context

9.3 How to Organize the Discussion

Start the discussion by first addressing the broader context of the study, drawing from existing literature and theoretical frameworks. Highlight what was found and how these findings contribute to the understanding of the topic and identify any gaps in the current research. As you examine further, focus specifically on the main findings, placing them within the context of what is already known. This can be thought of as an inverted pyramid, moving from general to specific.

Begin by describing the results and the significance of the main findings and then put them in perspective relative to what other researchers have discovered on the topic. This will help support the answers to the research questions and establish their relevance by comparing your findings with those from other studies. Conclude whether the results are similar or divergent from what has been previously reported in the literature. Discuss whether your findings align with or differ from the interpretations previously provided by other authors. Supporting these analyses with your results will provide a clearer understanding of the contributions your research makes. Consider potential alternative explanations for your findings and those observed by prior researchers. Understanding these perspectives is vital for comprehensive analysis. For a summary of the contents of the discussion section, see Box 9.1.

Box 9.1 Discussion Section

The discussion section should address and discuss:

- Describe the main results: what we found
- Attempt an explanation of those results
- Align with existing literature and studies
- Discuss what the results mean for clinical practice/policy making/future research
- Highlight limitations
- Make recommendations for further studies
- Conclusion:
  - Summarize, highlight unanswered questions and final thoughts

When developing the discussion, follow the same sequence as the study objectives presented earlier. For each objective or research question, directly mention the corresponding answer, without restating the question itself. This ensures clarity and coherence in your narrative. Extend the discussion using the same order of presentation in the results section, maintaining consistency with the material and methods sections. In terms of grammatical tense, stick to the present when interpreting results and discussing implications. For instance, “The average number of dental caries in the sample was…” (past tense) followed by “which is probably due to…” (present tense) will effectively communicate the findings and their implications.

Occasionally, remind the reader or reviewer of the research problem and the related questions being addressed, but avoid repetition. Introduce new points for discussion with contextual reminders or rephrasing that guide the reader to understand the focus of the upcoming analysis. Reference specific results but avoid excessive repetition of data. Instead, direct readers to relevant tables or figures for context.

Discuss the hypotheses generated from your findings, indicating that they should be tested and accepted or rejected in future studies with various designs or methodologies. Acknowledge the emergence of new research questions inspired by your results and suggest ways to pursue those inquiries. Consider recommending new populations, alternative research designs, or even qualitative methodologies, if appropriate, for deeper exploration.

Without a doubt, when reviewing a good manuscript, one can often find valuable suggestions on how to continue a line of research. Additionally, as emphasized in a previous chapter, conducting a comprehensive review of the literature before designing a research study is crucial. Such a review provides essential guidelines on which instruments or tools to use, what types of analysis are appropriate, and other relevant considerations. Incorporating these insights into the discussion section of the manuscript enhances the overall quality of the research. This information significantly aids researchers by offering a solid foundation for future studies.

As mentioned earlier, at the beginning of a study, researchers typically possess a general understanding of the topic and the existing body of knowledge. However, as the study progresses, the researcher becomes increasingly engaged with the subject, leading to a deeper comprehension. It is often only at the conclusion of the study that one fully grasps the complexities and nuances of the research topic. This reflection underscores the importance of recognizing one's starting point in the research journey, which ultimately forms part of the recommendations shared in the discussion section.

Before concluding or transitioning to the final section, it is imperative to identify the study's limitations and weaknesses. Every research endeavour possesses certain constraints related to design, sampling, or type of analysis, which should be presented truthfully as it is highly likely that reviewers will identify these shortcomings. By acknowledging the limitations inherent in our study, we demonstrate our awareness of their existence.

9.3.1 Lessons Learned

If mistakes are made, it is crucial to be forthright and clarify them. Clearly indicate any limitations that may pertain to the study, enabling future researchers to enhance their inquiry. Identifying these constraints contributes to the discourse by suggesting how a study might be conducted differently or explaining the reasons for such changes. Honesty is essential in conveying how these limitations may impact the validity of the findings. For instance, if one conducts a cross-sectional study or survey querying how many times a participant brushes their teeth daily, the most frequently reported answers will likely be "twice" or "three times", as these responses align with socially acceptable norms. Participants may not feel confident disclosing their true habits. It is vital to acknowledge that one limitation lies in the data being collected through self-reported surveys. Such an approach can potentially introduce bias to the results, since individuals may respond according to the social acceptability of their answers [1] which can skew the outcomes. Additionally, there are occasions when the required sample size was not achieved for various reasons, which affects our findings as a result. If this scenario applies, it should be addressed explicitly.

A cross-sectional study, for instance, cannot provide causation. This constitutes a limitation that must be acknowledged in the limitations section. Firstly, reviewers will undoubtedly detect it, and secondly, this type of acknowledgment offers insights into how to advance that line of inquiry, suggesting the next steps to pursue.

Nevertheless, it is essential to maintain honesty and self-critique without resorting to apologies. Rather, one should simply articulate the limitations of the study. Always take pride in your findings, because through identifying these limitations, you are proposing new perspectives on the issue at hand. Moreover, following the limitations section, it is prudent to articulate that, despite the acknowledged constraints of our study, its validity remains intact. Emphasize the value of the research, recognizing the limitations in design, analysis, and contextual circumstances. Indicate how the study's findings and conclusions are significant, bolstering a broader understanding of the research problem, which may subsequently lead to recommendations for future inquiries.

The summary should be the culmination of the discussion section. This may either be a distinct part of the discussion or integrated within it. Clearly outline the principal findings and connect them to the limitations previously discussed. In other words, it is crucial to recognize that the study had limitations, which may have influenced the results; however, considering these limitations, the study remains valid, as it offers fresh insights or new information on the topic we are investigating (e.g., the oral health of immigrants in Australia), especially considering the scarcity of existing knowledge.

We previously discussed that the organizational structure resembles an inverted pyramid, but towards the conclusion, we must once again broaden our scope. In essence, we begin with a generalization, and go into the specifics, and then examine how our precise findings bear relevance or validity in a more general context. Within the limitations of our study, the discussion should be structured to transition from the general to the specific, and then back to the general [2].

The length of this section follows the authors' guidelines. Typically, it is advisable that approximately one-third of the manuscript encompasses the introduction and methodology, another third is dedicated to the results, and the remaining third focuses on the discussion. It is crucial to remain creative, concise, and specific regarding word count and content inclusion, as not every finding can be accommodated in one manuscript. Research conducted by Bem found a correlation of –0.73 between the clarity of a researcher's results and the length of the discussion section, indicating that longer discussions often result in reduced clarity [3].

Occasionally, the discussion section may extend to encompass half of the manuscript because it serves as more than a discussion of the results. It can resemble an additional literature review. For instance, if one conducts a study on the prevalence of dental caries, there is no need to detail the process of caries development within the discussion. If this type of description were to be included, it would belong to the literature review. The discussion should focus on the results obtained and their significance within the context of the existing knowledge on the subject. Identifying unnecessary elements to be eliminated is, indeed, an art form.

9.4 Issues to Avoid

- Do not repeat the results. While it is acceptable to remind the reader of the topic being discussed, repeating results in detail is unnecessary. Instead, use bridging phrases to transition from the finding to its interpretation, and if needed, reference the table where the information is presented without going into specifics about values or statistical significance.
- Do not introduce new results in the discussion section; focus solely on the findings presented in the results section.
- Recommendations for future research should be included in either the discussion or the conclusion but avoid repeating the same ideas in both sections. It is often more appropriate to include them in the discussion, as many journals combine the conclusion with the discussion.
- The discussion should not be merely descriptive; it should include analysis rather than just reiterating the results.
- It is important to put the results into perspective by considering contributions from other authors. This should involve a deeper analysis rather than simply stating that the results are "similar to", "inferior to", or "superior to" previous studies. Elaborate on the comparisons made and explain why the findings result in such outcomes.
- When making comparisons, ensure they are relevant to the study and the context of your work. Of course, it depends on what is being discussed. But make sure the comparisons are relevant.
- Avoid overinterpreting the results and refrain from drawing conclusions that go beyond the study design. For instance, a cross-sectional study cannot establish causality; it can only suggest hypotheses related to cause and effect.
- Do not extend your analysis beyond what has been presented. If the study design involved is a bivariate analysis, do not come to conclusions that require a multivariate approach.

- Be cautious in not overinterpreting the findings, acknowledging that the sample size may limit the ability to make meaningful comparisons or generalizations due to inadequate statistical power or sampling characteristics.
- Exercise caution when generalizing results to other populations, as findings may not be applicable outside of the studied group.

When putting findings in context with other investigations, always do so with respect. If necessary, provide criticism of the research, but maintain respect for your fellow researchers. It is generally more effective to highlight the positive aspects of your own study and how it advances knowledge rather than focusing on criticizing others.

9.5 The Style

Style in scientific writing is inherently personal, and the general trend is to use the first-person plural for descriptions. The first-person singular should not be employed, even if the research is conducted by a single researcher. Instead, use either the first-person plural or impersonal language, such as "We discovered" or "The study discovered" or "It established". Using the first person does not undermine the scientific validity of the results, but it can distract the reader or reviewer from the findings you wish to convey.

Engaging in peer review within the research team is crucial and all authors and co-authors should participate in this process. When you are engrossed in the preparation of an article, certain details might be overlooked, but having colleagues review the work decreases the likelihood of this.

9.6 The Qualitative Manuscript

The structure of a qualitative manuscript differs from that of a quantitative one in that the results section typically combines results and discussion. There is also a discussion section in qualitative manuscripts; however, it is generally shorter and serves more as a conclusion than a comprehensive analysis. It can be much briefer than the discussion in a quantitative manuscript. The conclusions drawn should align with the themes and topics presented in the introduction. Consistency is key, meaning that everything must relate to the questions posed initially. In the discussion, it is important not to simply repeat what has already been stated in the text. Rather, focus on analysing, dissecting, and providing thoughtful insights into the content.

9.7 Summary

- The discussion section should progress from the general to the specific then back to the general.
- Be concise, brief, and specific.
- Support arguments with the data obtained and existing literature.
- Discuss findings in relation to the research question.
- Avoid presenting new findings or discussing results that were not included in the results section.
- Discuss and appraise conflicting results, especially if there is a discrepancy between existing literature and your findings. Discuss the possible reasons for this.
- Discuss and evaluate unexpected findings, exploring why they occurred.
- Present relationships with the existing literature and the generalizations that can be drawn from the results.
- Indicate the implications of your study and its potential practical applications. Acknowledge the limitations of the study openly, as they are likely to be apparent to many readers.

There is some debate regarding whether limitations should be introduced at the beginning or towards the end of the discussion section; I recommend positioning them towards the end, followed by a paragraph emphasizing the study's findings, stating that despite these limitations, the study remains valid for specific reasons, for example the sample size or geographical context, etc.

- Include suggestions for future research regarding aspects such as sample selection, types of analysis, research methodology (e.g., qualitative or quantitative), instruments to utilize, and variables to include. Remember, by the conclusion of the study, you will have a clearer understanding of how the research should have originally been conducted.
- Above all, refrain from including conclusions that could have been drawn without data from the study; do not make assertions that could have been made without conducting the research.

9.8 Writing the Conclusions Section

As previously mentioned, certain journals request a conclusion separate from the discussion section. This section is typically shorter than the previous ones. There can be various formats, with some journals asking for a bullet-point summary of the key points. Regardless of whether it is included as a separate section or as part of the discussion, this section serves a very specific purpose and function.

Its objective is to emphasize the significance of the research being reported. It presents the final opportunity to stress why the results, the findings, and the research matter. This message succinctly condenses what the reader should remember from the study, serving as a takeaway or lasting impression. This enduring impression is achieved by highlighting the most important aspects of the findings or the analysis performed. Therefore, do not hesitate to highlight the importance of your study, referring to the novel detail or insight generated through the research that the reader should retain. However, one must not go beyond the limitations of what the data can support.

If the journal does not feature a separate conclusions section, include a final paragraph towards the conclusion of the discussion, which would fulfil the role of the conclusion, albeit not as a separate section. This depends on the format stipulated by the journal to which you are submitting the manuscript.

Regardless of the format, it is vital to succinctly summarize the thoughts of the author or authors and the implications of the study towards practical applications in health policy, new investigative methods, or alternative ways of addressing a problem. Remember, this should be done in a very concise and summarized manner, emphasizing not only the new findings but also new approaches to thinking about or examining a research problem.

9.8.1 Some Considerations When Writing the Conclusion Section

- Generally, the conclusions are presented as a single paragraph, though multiple paragraphs can be used if necessary. The most important aspect is to ensure that the writing is clear and straightforward. In this paragraph, emphasize what is novel and highlight the contribution to knowledge. Therefore, it should not merely summarize the results or the study; but must also stress the new points.
- The conclusion serves as the final opportunity to position a specific finding within a broader context, but it should not extend beyond the limits of the data.
- It is acceptable to indicate new lines of research that emerge in this final paragraph. However, remember that if this was already addressed in the discussion, repetition is unnecessary, but if not mentioned in the discussion, this is an opportunity to include it.
- Keep in mind the pyramid structure of the discussion, transitioning from the specific to the general should form the conclusion or the final segment of the discussion. The specific results need to be presented within a broader context,

addressing their utility. For example, articulate how a specific finding might benefit a health program, or contribute to broader health policies, or an emerging line of research, such as a new methodology being presented. (Formatting)
- The conclusion or final part of the discussion must be consistent and aligned to the objectives. If the objectives and conclusions are not in sync, there is a problem.
- Avoid concluding on matters that could have been inferred without conducting the study. It is all too common to see conclusions drawn about unrelated issues. Therefore, do not use those precious few closing words on something that was already known.
- This is different from placing findings within a broader context—always ensure that your findings are contextualized.
- The conclusions must be supported by the evidence presented in the study and by existing literature.

9.8.2 Issues to Avoid When Writing the Conclusions Section

- Being verbose and failing to be concise.
- Not providing a clear summary of the new information being presented.
- Lack of commentary on broader significant issues, such as health policies, education, or other research areas.
- Neglecting to mention any negative results. There is a tendency towards reporting only the statistically significant findings, overlooking any non-significant results that may still be information or unique innovations in their own right.
- Controversial results can also contribute valuable insights into a topic.
- Failing to fulfil the objectives of the research.
- Not supporting conclusions with evidence.
- In the conclusions or closing statements:
  - Emphasizing what is novel.
  - Defining unanswered questions or providing recommendations for future research.
  - Going beyond the limitations of the data.

This chapter incorporates practical activities (see Activity 9.1 and Activity 9.2 in the Appendix), which engage the readers in practical applications of the concepts and knowledge included in the chapter to prepare them for real-world applications in their area of interest.

Appendix

Activity 9.1	
1) Describe what the new knowledge(s) acquired is. Write your answer here: a. Research question 1. ____________ ____________ b. Research question 2. ____________ ____________ c. Research question 3. ____________ ____________	
2) Describe what the next step(s) might be? Write your answer here: ____________ ____________ ____________ ____________	
3) Checklist:	
a. Presents what the new knowledge. If "No", how can I improve this aspect? ____________ ____________	**Yes No**
b. Presents the results from general to specific. If "No", how can I improve this aspect? ____________ ____________	**Yes No**
c. Have you included discussion of the results that answer its research questions. If "No", how can I improve this aspect? ____________ ____________	**Yes No**
d. Have you interpreted the results in the light of existing knowledge. Link your findings to the literature. If "No", how can I improve this aspect? ____________ ____________	**Yes No**

(continued)

(continued)

e. Have you provided a subjective or speculative interpretation of the meaning of the results. If "No", how can I improve this aspect? ________________ ________________	**Yes No**
f. Has provided a subjective or speculative interpretation of the meaning of the results. If "No", how can I improve this aspect? ________________ ________________	**Yes No**
g. Have you described whether each hypothesis was supported or refuted. If "No", how can I improve this aspect? ________________ ________________	**Yes No**
h. Connects, but does not repeat, the introduction If "No", how can I improve this aspect? ________________ ________________	**Yes No**
i. Presents new findings or discusses results not presented in the results. If "No", how can I improve this aspect? ________________ ________________	**Yes No**
j. Does identify limitations and weaknesses. If "No", how can I improve this aspect? ________________ ________________	**Yes No**
k. Does link your findings to theory. If "No", how can I improve this aspect? ________________ ________________	**Yes No**
l. Does link your findings to practice. If "No", how can I improve this aspect? ________________ ________________	**Yes No**

(continued)

(continued)

Activity 9.2
1) Do the conclusions address the objective/research question/hypothesis? Describe what the conclusion is for each research question. Write your answer here: a. Conclusion research question 1. ______________________ ______________________ b. Conclusion research question 2. ______________________ ______________________ c. Conclusion research question n. ______________________ ______________________

References

1. Sackett DL. Bias in analytic research. J Chronic Dis. 1979;32:51–63. https://doi.org/10.1016/0021-9681(79)90012-2.
2. Sacred Heart University. Research guides: organizing academic research papers: 8. The discussion. Sacred Hearth University. Library. 2013. https://library.sacredheart.edu/c.php?g=29803&p=185933. Accessed 18 Nov 2024.
3. Bem DJ. Writing the empirical journal article. In: Darley JM, Zanna MP, Roediger HL, editors. The compleat academic: A career guide. 2nd ed. Washington, DC: American Psychological Association; 2004. p. 185–219.

Chapter 10
Preparation of an Original Article: Abstract Preparation, Keywords, and Management of Bibliographical References

Ebingen Villavicencio-Caparó and Rodrigo Mariño

10.1 Introduction

The goal of the abstract is, as the name suggests, to summarize an article and allow the reader, reviewer, or examiner to get a quick overview of the study and decide whether they want to read/review/examine the work itself. However, for a peer reviewer and an examiner, once the task is accepted, they do not have to decide whether they are going to continue reading the article, or the entire thesis, because they have already committed to doing so. However, the abstract is important because that reviewer or examiner will be selected based on its content. That is, the type of information and the objectives indicated in the abstract will determine their selection.

In general, the reader, as a consumer of information, is the one who selects an article based on the information contained in the abstract. Therefore, as previously mentioned in Chap. 6 the abstract might be the last thing that is written, however it is crucial because it will define many relevant outcomes for the article or the thesis. There is a phrase often attributed to Oscar Wilde: "*You never get a second chance to*

E. Villavicencio-Caparó (✉)
Universidad Católica de Cuenca, Cuenca, Ecuador

Universidad Peruana Cayetano Heredia, Lima, Perú
e-mail: evillavicencioc@ucacue.edu.ec

R. Mariño
Melbourne Dental School, The University of Melbourne, Melbourne, Australia

Center for Research in Epidemiology, Economics and Oral Public Health (CIEESPO), University de la Frontera, Temuco, Chile

Department of Conservative Dentistry and Oral Health, Riga Stradins University, Riga, Latvia

Monash Health Dental Services, Melbourne, Australia
e-mail: r.marino@unimelb.edu.au

R. Mariño et al. (eds.), *Scientific Writing and Publication Strategies for Oral Health Professionals*, https://doi.org/10.1007/978-3-031-97916-3_10

make a first impression" and this is what an abstract does, it creates a first impression that encourages the reader to continue. Thus, it is our opportunity to make a good impression.

In addition to making a good impression, the importance of the abstract lies in its incorporation or indexing in databases, such as Medline, where researchers and those seeking specific information and evidence will access it. First, they will see the title and then they will read the abstract. Consequently, keywords are as important as the abstract, because searches are primarily conducted through keywords. If they are not carefully selected, our study may not appear in as many search results. What we want is exposure; thus, the significance of the title, abstract, and keywords is essential for the manuscript's visibility.

Furthermore, librarians use abstracts to highlight articles in library newsletters and on digital resource platforms, which increases the visibility of key scientific publications and facilitates access to relevant research for their user community [1]. The abstract also aids researchers in constructing a theoretical framework to quickly identify the value and usefulness of a paper, allowing them to engage in further reading if deemed appropriate, or to discard it if it does not meet their aims.

As mentioned in Chap. 6, these three elements (the title, the abstract, and the keywords) are finalized at the end of our study. This is because it is only at that moment, after having worked for a year or more on a topic, that the researcher gains a deeper understanding of the material. Moreover, after the manuscript or final report has been written, the researcher is better placed to identify the key aspects and most important elements of the study.

10.2 The Abstract

10.2.1 Historical Development

The creation of the abstract in scientific research is a practice that has evolved throughout the history of scientific knowledge. Its purpose is to condense the essential information of a study and facilitate quick understanding and communication of the findings to other researchers.

According to Robert Day, the first scientific journals appeared in France and in England in 1665. Summarizing an academic work is a practice that has its origins in the Renaissance (fifteenth to eighteenth centuries) and began to develop along with the proliferation of scientific publications from the seventeenth century onward [2]. Many books and articles on scientific discoveries grew during the Renaissance and the Enlightenment, leading to the need to condense information for a wider audience. This custom was on the rise by the nineteenth century, and the term "abstract" was formalized, which synthesizes the aims, methods, results, and conclusions of an article. This type of abstract helped researchers decide whether the content of an article was relevant to their studies [3]. With the expansion of science and technology post World War II, scientific publishing experienced exponential growth. Competition for a scoop in the publication of scientific findings and the need to disseminate information quickly to gain academic prestige made the abstract standard in all scientific articles. With the advent of digital databases and online repositories, the abstract has become even more important, as it is used as a tool for indexing and finding articles in academic search engines.

Abstracts of scientific research are very useful tools for librarians because they facilitate the indexing and location of information. They are a resource that serves to quickly assess the relevance and quality of an article and decide whether it should be included in a specific collection or recommended to library users [4].

10.2.2 Technical Issues

Generally, during submission, the abstract is uploaded in a separate page from the main manuscript. In some journals, it is uploaded as a separate file. That is, you submit the abstract in a different section to the main files. Other times, the abstract must also be incorporated into the article itself. This is why it is important to always read the instructions for authors carefully, otherwise, the manuscript may be returned within a few hours for not placing the title, abstract, or keywords in the correct sections.

10.2.3 Abstracts Structure

There are two types of abstracts: structured and unstructured. We emphasize the need to follow the journal's instructions for the type of abstract required.

10.2.3.1 Structured Abstracts

Structured abstracts generally replicate, in a condensed format, the IMRaD (Introduction, Materials and Methods, Results, and Discussion) structure of the article sections, with separate headings for each.

10.2.3.2 Unstructured Abstracts

Unstructured abstracts do not have specific indications regarding the parts they should contain. Readers will still identify the objective of the study, materials and methods, results, and conclusions when reading the abstract, but without headings to guide them.

10.2.4 Word Limits

The length of the abstract varies depending on the journal (i.e., follow the instructions). Commonly, abstracts range between 250 and 350 words, but they may also exceed 400, or be as short as 50 words. Authors must carefully select phrases, words, or information to include in the abstract, summarizing up to 2 or 3 years of research in a concise format. Abstracts are usually written as a single paragraph, so it is crucial to ensure that there are no contradictions or redundancies in relation to the rest of the manuscript.

10.2.4.1 Content

Since the summary must be brief, it should not contain more than:

Introduction or Context Starts with the formulation of the problem or an indication of its context, clearly stating the main question or the purpose of the research. It should include the objective, as found in the introduction. Sometimes, abstract guidelines may request background and supporting information, while other times they may start directly with the objective or purpose of the research. In this case, clearly state the primary objectives of the study, specifying what it aims to achieve or discover [5].

When writing this section, you need to construct a phrase that summarizes these elements in the problem formulation. Include:

- A brief explanation of the research topic, its relevance, and the problem addressed by the study, providing insight into the long-term purpose of the research. It is recommended to keep this section concise and focused, avoiding any excessive detail or unnecessary information. Present only the essentials to ensure that the reader quickly understands what aspect of general knowledge the research topic pertains to [6].

  Identify the problem that the research addresses or the central question that the study seeks to answer, establishing its relevance. Provide only the necessary information about previous studies or the current state of knowledge in the field. This might include one or two sentences that highlight a literature gap or justify the study's need, conveying why it is relevant to address this problem or question. Discuss the potential impact of the research, which may include practical clinical, theoretical, or social implications.

  To make the abstract engaging from the start, it is a good idea to use terms relevant to the field of study [7]. This approach helps readers quickly identify research topics and assists academic search engines in accurately indexing articles. The abstract is usually written in the past tense, unless indicated otherwise in the author's guide [8].

Methodology or Materials and Methods Includes a succinct description of the study design, sample size, data collection methods, and analysis techniques [9, 10]. Due to the limited space available for the abstract, it is impossible to include all of the technical details; only enough information should be provided for the reader to understand how the study was conducted. Begin by mentioning the design of the study and then describe the characteristics of the sample or study participants, including the number of participants. Next, highlight essential methods used to collect the data, for example, observations, interviews, surveys, etc.

A concise sentence indicating the statistical or analytical methods used to interpret the data helps to add weight to an abstract [10]. It is not necessary to include technical details such as specific procedural steps or equipment configurations, unless they are critical to understanding the results. Technical terms should be used appropriately so that non-specialist readers can understand the basic methodology. Finally, specify the place and time in which the variables were measured, especially in studies involving human subjects.

Results A summary of the most relevant results should be provided without excessive detail. These findings are derived from the results section of the manuscript, but again, it is important not to include everything. Avoid minor details that are not essential to the overall understanding of the study [11]. Focus on the finding that directly answers the main research question. It is advisable to provide specific figures such as percentages, means, and confidence intervals to enhance the precision and persuasiveness of the results, helping readers understand the importance of the observed effects.

The presentation of results in the abstract should concentrate on what was found, rather than the implications of those findings [12]. Interpretation of the results should be left for the conclusions section of the abstract or discussion section of the article [13]. However, it should be kept in mind that the abstract should not include extensive details of all results, only the most relevant ones.

Conclusions A conclusion is fundamental to any research work, so it should be explicitly included in the abstract. It should provide a brief interpretation of the results and their significance in relation to the study's objectives [14]. The conclusion may also highlight implications, recommendations, or the relevance of the findings in terms of future research. Ideally, it should be separate from the results and may consist of one or two sentences that derive from the discussion section of the manuscript or from its conclusion section, if one exists.

The conclusion represents the closure of the study and aims to synthesize the results obtained, answer the research questions posed, and reflect on the implications and significance of these findings. While it can be slightly extended to indicate trends identified during the research, this will depend on the word limit allowed for the abstract. Importantly, conclusions should not be drawn that could have been reached without conducting this research. They should directly reference the results and emphasize what is unique about the research conducted.

Each element of the abstract, the objective, the methodology, the results and the conclusions must be consistent. The reader should be able to understand the content of the abstract without needing to reference the manuscript itself. Moreover, avoid concluding with statements like: "*further research is needed,*" as this is an obvious assertion applicable to any study. Instead, use the limited word count of the abstract to indicate, for example, what type of research could be conducted in the future.

You could also indicate that the study has some limitations, but this should be done concisely, usually in one or two sentences. Do not include conclusions that extend beyond the results presented in the abstract.

10.2.5 Problems to Avoid

When you finish the abstract, ask yourself: if that were the only accessible part of the document or manuscript, would you be satisfied with the amount of information presented? Are you content with the message conveyed in the abstract? If your answers are: "No," perhaps it may be necessary to review and reconsider the information being provided. However, be critical in your assessment and do not treat it as a mere task to tick off. Remember that, for example in a systematic literature review, the selection of articles will be based on the keywords, the title, and the abstract.

The chapter includes a practical activity (see Activity 10.1 in the Appendix) with a step-by-step guide designed to be applied in a real-world situation relevant to the readers' area of interest.

10.2.5.1 General Recommendations

- Some abstract guidelines do not allow for a background section and start directly with the objectives. If you have background information include it, but avoid excessive detail to prevent taking words away from the results, which should highlight the novel aspects of your study.
- In general, abstracts do not use references, but this applies only to the abstract and not to the manuscript itself.
- Avoid using ellipses or incomplete sentences. While we can often imply meaning in spoken language, the abstract requires clarity as the reader may not understand its meaning without full sentences.
- Do not use abbreviations or terms that may confuse the reader, as they may have different meanings in various contexts (e.g., DMF or CPI could have different meanings depending on the profession and context).

- Typically, images, figures, tables, etc. are not included in the abstract. Additionally, do not refer to tables present in the manuscript, since the reader or the reviewer may not have direct access to those tables.
- If the abstract is structured, use subheadings to delineate each section of the abstract clearly.

10.3 Keywords

Keywords are a list of terms that represent the main concepts of the study. The importance of keywords is that they define the field or topic of research. This helps the indexing and retrieval of the research in academic databases, which were explained in depth in Chap. 3. For this reason, it is important to look for the words that describe the study, which are usually predefined.

These keywords also play a role in the selection of manuscript reviewers and determining the appropriate section of the journal for publication, or even the journal itself out of several options that a publisher might have. Additionally, for research proposals, the keywords will determine who will review the proposal. Therefore, the selection of keywords is crucial not only for the initial submission, but also for the future visibility and impact of the manuscript or research proposal.

Many journals utilize headings of medical terms from the National Library of Medicine in the USA, managed by PubMed or Medline, which include a section of Medical Subject headings (MeSH). Authors should search for these terms to ensure consistency with these themes. Generally, journals request between three and five keywords, so it is essential to check the specific requirements of the selected journal. Additionally, verify whether the journal allows authors to create new keywords, as this policy may vary. Some journals provide a restricted menu of terms to choose from.

Another suggestion would be not to use the same words as the title. This gives authors a better chance of a researcher identifying the article.

For example, when selecting keywords for a study on chemical-mechanical caries removal, it is essential to capture the procedure's essence while attracting broader research on related topics. Key terms like "chemical-mechanical caries removal" clearly identify the study's focus, while terms like "minimally invasive dentistry" and "caries treatment alternatives" broaden its reach to similar studies in the field. Using specific phrases like "caries lesion softening agents" further narrows the scope to the chemicals used in the process. The goal is to make the study easily discoverable by those researching both specific aspects of caries removal and other related topics.

10.3.1 How to Select Keywords

To select keywords in MeSH for an article about caries and risk factors, follow these steps to ensure accuracy and consistency:

10.3.1.1 Access the MeSH Database in PubMed

Search in the browser MESH or PubMed and select "MeSH Database." The MeSH database provides a list of standardized terms that describe specific concepts in biomedicine and public health.

10.3.1.2 Search for the Main Term

Type the main term of the study, for example, "Caries" or "Dental Caries," in the MeSH search bar. The database will display the corresponding term in MeSH, such as "Dental Caries," which is the correct descriptor for the topic of dental caries.

10.3.1.3 Explore Subcategories or Related Terms

Click on the main term ("Dental Caries") and review the subcategories and related terms, such as "Tooth Demineralization" or "Tooth Diseases." You can choose those terms that best represent specific aspects of your research.

10.3.1.4 Use the MeSH Hierarchy to Refine Specificity

The hierarchical structure of MeSH allows you to select more specific (descending) or more general (ascending) terms within the same concept. This allows you to opt for broad or detailed keywords depending on your search objective. For example, if your focus is very specific, you could select "Cariogenic Agents" [MeSH] instead of "Diet, Cariogenic."

10.3.1.5 Check Consistency and Add Keywords to the Abstract

Review the selected keywords to make sure they cover all the main aspects of your research. Add them to the article abstract in a format similar to:

Keywords: Dental Caries; Risk Factors; Oral Hygiene; Cariogenic Diet; Socioeconomic Factors.

10.4 Management of Bibliographical References

Another activity that should be carried out in the final stages of preparing a manuscript is adapting the bibliographic references to the author's standards outlined by the journal. This process will not only ensure that references are presented in a consistent format, but also enhance the professionalism and credibility of the work.

Different journals may adhere to various citation styles, such as APA, MLA, Chicago, or other guidelines unique to their publishing policy. Adhering to these standards is essential, as it demonstrates the author's attention to detail and respect for academic integrity. Furthermore, accurately formatted references enable readers to locate the original sources, fostering transparency and facilitating further research. Inconsistent or improperly formatted citations can lead to confusion, diminish the perceived quality of the manuscript, and potentially result in rejection during the peer-review process. By ensuring that bibliographic references are meticulously adjusted according to the journal's specifications, authors enhance the accessibility and visibility of their work within the academic community.

Use of one of the bibliographic managers listed in Table 10.1 is recommended for this purpose:

The general process used for the management of bibliographic references with referencing software is:

- Installation of the software or application.
- Location of the document to be referenced in physical, PDF, or website.
- Identify the text to be cited (textual quotation or paraphrase).
- Write the text in the article, and the author's citation located in the previous steps at the end of the paragraph.
- Upload the document to the reference software. This will automatically recognize the metadata of the document and offer a report indicating its title and author; if this information coincides with the document to be cited, click on the add citation button. The author's last name and year of publication will appear in the word processor.
- After adding the last citation, the reference software is asked to update the citations and bibliography so that the bibliographic references appear at the document's end.

Table 10.1 Bibliography managers

Software	Description	Characteristics	Platforms	License
EndNote	Complete program for reference management with advanced organization and citation tools	Integration with Word, PDF storage, advanced search, cloud synchronization	Windows, macOS	Paid
Mendeley	Free reference manager that also functions as an academic social network	Integration with Word and LibreOffice, cloud storage, collaborative work	Windows, macOS, Linux, iOS, Android	Free (paid options available)
Zotero	Free and open-source tool for reference management	Browser extension, integration with Word, Google Docs and LibreOffice, PDF support, group work	Windows, macOS, Linux	Free
RefWorks	Web-based reference manager focused on writing and collaboration	Integration with Word and Google Docs, data import/export, collaboration, cloud storage	Web	Paid
Citavi	Reference and knowledge manager with tools for project planning and organization	Integration with Word, idea organization, text annotation, task planning	Windows	Paid (limited free version)
Papers	Reference and scientific literature management tool designed for science researchers	Integration with Word, database search, PDF annotation, device synchronization	Windows, macOS, iOS	Paid
JabRef	Open-source reference manager based on BibTeX, mainly for LaTeX users	Integration with LaTeX, reference organization, format support, online search	Windows, macOS, Linux	Free
Cite This For Me	Online tool that allows generating citations in multiple styles	Automatic citation generator, user-friendly interface, multiple style support, project saving	Web	Free (paid options available)
BibDesk	macOS application designed to manage bibliographies and references, especially for LaTeX users	Integration with BibTeX, reference search, citation organization	macOS	Free
Paperpile	Cloud-based reference manager designed to integrate perfectly with Google Docs and Drive	Direct integration with Google Docs and Google Drive, automatic cloud sync, PDF search and management, citation generation	Web, Chrome extension, iOS, Android	Paid with a 30-day free trial

Appendix

Activity 10.1 Preparing your abstract
1) Write the objective/purpose of your research Write your answer here: ____________________ ____________________ ____________________ ____________________
2) Write down your research methodology Write your answer here: ____________________ ____________________ ____________________ ____________________
3) Write the results of your research Write your answer here: ____________________ ____________________ ____________________ ____________________
4) Write the results of your research Write your answer here: ____________________ ____________________ ____________________ ____________________
5) Write the conclusion(s) of your research Write your answer here: ____________________ ____________________ ____________________ ____________________
6) Write down the implications of your research Write your answer here: ____________________ ____________________ ____________________ ____________________

References

1. Spicer S. Exploring video abstracts in science journals: An overview and case study. J Libr Sch Commun. 2014;2(2):1110. https://doi.org/10.7710/2162-3309.1110.
2. Day R, Gastel B. How to write and publish a scientific paper. 7th ed. Santa Barbara: Greenwood; 2011.
3. Bazerman C. Shaping written knowledge: the genre and activity of the experimental article in science. Madison: University of Wisconsin Press; 1988.
4. Blobaum P. Abstracts and abstracting: a genre and set of skills for the twenty-first century. J Med Libr Assoc. 2012;100:324. https://doi.org/10.3163/1536-5050.100.4.020.
5. Hawhee V. How to build an abstract. J Registry Manag. 2016;43:42–3.
6. Drury A, Pape E, Dowling M, Miguel S, Fernández-Ortega P, Papadopoulou C, Kotronoulas G. How to write a comprehensive and informative research abstract. Semin Oncol Nurs. 2023;39:151395. https://doi.org/10.1016/j.soncn.2023.151395.
7. Kaspersen AE, Hasenkam JM, Leipziger JG, Djurhuus JC. [Introduction on how to write a scientific abstract]. Ugeskr Laeger. 2019;181:V02190103.
8. Kallet RH. How to write the methods section of a research paper. Respir Care. 2004;49:1229–32.
9. Mattick K, Johnston J, de la Croix A. How to…write a good research question. Clin Teach. 2018;15:104–8. https://doi.org/10.1111/tct.12776.
10. Meade MH, Michael M, Henzes J, Nanavati R, Woods B. How to write an abstract. Clin Spine Surg. 2024; https://doi.org/10.1097/BSD.0000000000001667.
11. Dhillon P. How to write a good scientific review article. FEBS J. 2022;289:3592–602. https://doi.org/10.1111/febs.16565.
12. Alexandrov A. How to write a research paper. Cerebrovasc Dis. 2024;18(2):135–8. https://doi.org/10.1159/000079266.
13. Snyder N, Foltz C, Lendner M, Vaccaro AR. How to write an effective results section. Clin Spine Surg. 2019;32:295–6. https://doi.org/10.1097/BSD.0000000000000845.
14. Makar G, Foltz C, Lendner M, Vaccaro AR. How to write effective discussion and conclusion sections. Clin Spine Surg. 2018;31:345–6. https://doi.org/10.1097/BSD.0000000000000687.

Chapter 11
Article Submission Strategy

Rodrigo Mariño

11.1 Introduction

Lately, with the due to an increase in online publications and open-access journals, there has been an expansion of publication possibilities in academic journals. This has significantly transformed the scientific publishing landscape, offering researchers more options to disseminate their research findings. However, this diversity also creates the need for careful evaluation of which journal the manuscript will be submitted to. By doing this, researchers can maximize the dissemination and impact of their work in the academic community.

Selecting the appropriate journal for manuscript submission is a multi-faceted decision that requires researchers to carefully weigh up various factors. Through conducting a thorough review of aspects such as the journal scope, reputation, peer-review processes, open-access options, and publication guidelines, authors can effectively enhance the visibility and impact of their research within the academic community. This informed and strategic approach to journal selection ultimately reinforces the significance of the scholarly work and contributes to the advancement of knowledge in a specific field. Therefore, this decision is crucial in the publication process and must be approached seriously and with meticulous attention. In order to do this, it is essential to consider several factors that can influence the visibility and impact of the work.

R. Mariño (✉)
Melbourne Dental School, The University of Melbourne, Melbourne, Australia

Center for Research in Epidemiology, Economics and Oral Public Health (CIEESPO), University de la Frontera, Temuco, Chile

Department of Conservative Dentistry and Oral Health, Riga Stradins University, Riga, Latvia

Monash Health Dental Services, Melbourne, Australia
e-mail: r.marino@unimelb.edu.au

R. Mariño et al. (eds.), *Scientific Writing and Publication Strategies for Oral Health Professionals*, https://doi.org/10.1007/978-3-031-97916-3_11

11.2 How to Select Journal

Selecting the appropriate journal for your manuscript is a critical step in publication process. Below are important considerations and steps to guide you in selecting the right journal [1–5]:

11.2.1 Objectives of the Journal

When selecting a journal, review the theme and objectives of the journal and make sure that they are consistent with the type of study that is being prepared. It is essential to verify whether the journal's focus is on accordance with the theme of your manuscript before submission.

11.2.2 Manuscript Type

Authors should verify what type of manuscripts are typically published by the journal. There are several possibilities, including quantitative or qualitative research, literature reviews, editorials, letters to the editor, case reports, opinion pieces, etc. Some journals may only accept original research manuscripts and may not consider literature reviews. Therefore, always review the specific types of manuscripts that the journal accepts.

This can be also done by examining the journal's index and analysing the manuscripts published in recent issues. Such an assessment will provide insights into the kinds of submissions the journal is currently accepting.

Another option is to contact the journal's editor directly. You can send the editor your abstract and the title of your manuscript to see whether it fits within the journal's publication guidelines. However, even if the editor indicates that the topic aligns with the journal's focus, this does not guarantee acceptance at the end of the review process. It does, nonetheless, provide some guidance, as editors typically respond positively to such requests, reflecting the collaborative relationship between authors and editors [6].

11.2.3 Impact Factor

An important factor to investigate is the impact factor of the journal, which indicates how often the journal is cited. Many universities place significant emphasis on the impact factor when evaluating academic publications for promotion purposes. Publishing in a high-impact journal can increase visibility and prestige; however, the competition for publication in these journals can be intense. High-impact journals often have a more rigorous review process, potentially decreasing acceptance rates [6]. For instance, in the Journal of Dental Research (JDR), approximately 50% of submitted manuscripts do not progress to peer review [7]. Nonetheless, a rigorous and transparent review process enhances the quality of the publication and strengthens the credibility of the results presented [8].

11.2.4 The Editorial Board of the Journal

It is also important to check the composition of the journal's editorial board. Typically, indexed journals have an editorial board, and reviewing its members can give you a sense of the journal's academic integrity and focus. Knowing who is on the board may provide insights into the journal's reputation and whether it aligns with your field of research.

11.2.5 The Journal's Target Audience

Authors should investigate the reach and audience of the journal in relation to the intended target audience of their manuscript. Consider which audience the authors aim to reach and determine who would find the information the most useful, necessary, or valuable. It is crucial to recognize that the manuscript's target audience may be local rather than the international. Researchers often aim for those involved in developing health policy or programs to access this information in order to facilitate new initiatives. Therefore, the manuscript should be published in a journal that this audience can access and in a language they understand.

11.2.6 Journal Peer-Review Policy

The journal's peer-review policy is another critical element to consider. Authors should also review the journal's open-access policies (see Sect. 11.2.12), deciding whether they wish their work to be accessible to the general public, or if they prefer a subscription-based model.

11.2.7 Publication Times

Authors should evaluate the publication timelines established by the journal, including publication rates and any specific formatting requirements. When selecting the journal, it is important to check if the system allows for transfers to other journals.

This occurs when a manuscript is rejected—some journals offer the option to transfer the manuscript to another journal within the same publishing house.

11.2.8 Number of Words, Tables, and Figures

Another factor to consider is the word limit imposed by different journals. For example, qualitative research or literature reviews generally require more words than manuscripts reporting quantitative research. If the chosen journal has a strict word limit, the manuscript may be rejected for exceeding it, or the authors may be asked to reduce the word count. The same consideration applies to the number of images, figures, and tables allowed.

While online publications tend to be less restrictive regarding word counts, with no additional cost for extra pages, traditional print journals usually have tighter limits. Authors should be aware that going beyond the allowed number of pages may result in a charge for the additional material, so it is essential to confirm whether the journal charges a fee for extra pages, as outlined in the authors' instructions.

11.2.9 Website

Check whether the journal has a dedicated website and evaluate its quality. Generally, journals provide an online platform where authors can enter their details, including names, abstracts, and keywords. This website serves as an interface for authors to populate various sections of the manuscript.

11.2.10 Indexing

Another matter to determine is whether the journal is indexed, as not all journals are. If the journal is indexed, identify which databases it is included in. This information is typically available on the journal's website. Indexed journals appear in databases where researchers can find articles relevant to their topic. (ref. think, check, and submit). Examples of recognized databases include:

- *PubMed*: free access.
- *SciELO*: focused on Latin America.
- *Latindex*: a Spanish-language resource that includes magazines from Latin America, the Caribbean, Spain, and Portugal.
- *Scopus*: a multidisciplinary database.
- *Web of Science*: subscription service.

11.2.11 Tools Available for Authors

Authors can evaluate the types of tools and resources that the journal provides to facilitate publication. Some journals may, for instance, offer editing support including assistance with writing the manuscript. Additionally, if the authors are not native speakers of the journal's language, services such as language review, translation, and English correction may be available, usually for a fee.

11.2.12 Open Access and Publication Costs

Choosing between open-access journals and subscription-only journals is another critical factor to consider. Open-access journals allow any reader to access articles online without restrictions, while subscription journals limit access to subscribers. Many universities maintain subscriptions to various journals, enabling their members to freely access published content. However, authors need to consider the publication costs and the open-access model when deciding where to submit their manuscript.

It is important to check for any costs associated with publication, commonly referred to as Article Processing Charges (APC). This cost has become standard practice, where authors are responsible for covering the administrative expenses related to the manuscript, peer-review process, and final publication. This information should be clearly detailed in the journal's instructions to authors.

11.2.13 Publication Language

The publication language may also be an important consideration, particularly in determining whether the target audience of your manuscript can effectively make use of the information presented.

Taking all these factors into account can greatly assist in choosing an appropriate journal for the publication of your manuscript. Some journals are more frequently used by researchers in your field, so it is crucial to evaluate the prestige and scientific standing of the journal, the qualifications of its editorial board members, and the overall quality of its website.

11.3 Publication Ethics

First and foremost, authors must submit the manuscript to only one journal at a time. Many journals will inquire during the submission process whether the manuscript has been submitted to any other journal and honesty in this regard is imperative. Although it may be difficult to verify, it reflects an ethical issue. Most reviewers are volunteers and submitting to more than one journal duplicates the number of reviewers who will invest their time reviewing the article and providing feedback. Therefore, submitting to multiple journals is a misuse of the process, as only one journal can continue the publication process to its conclusion.

Moreover, another unethical situation arises when some authors submit the same manuscript with different author lists to different journals, or when near-identical manuscripts are sent to various journals under different authorship. This is a clear violation of publication ethics.

To ensure that these rules are upheld, various resources have been developed, such as "Think, Check, Submit" [4]. In some cases, a journal publishes a manuscript, only for it to be retracted after identification of issues regarding its originality. Certain organizations also exist to review and monitor compliance, although such violations can still occur.

Publication ethics also extend to authorship. Only individuals who genuinely contributed to the creation of the article should be included as authors or co-authors. Including non-legitimate authors can inflate their h-index and perhaps their academic standing, but this is unethical and constitutes fraud.

As outlined in Chap. 2, a manuscript presents the results of an investigation that is both original and reflective of the authors' contributions. While the paper is grounded in the authors' own insights, it also incorporates other concepts derived from various sources. The use of others' ideas, expressions, or phrases whilst pretending that they reflect our own thoughts, without acknowledgment, whether through negligence or deliberate intent, is recognized as a serious ethical violation known as "plagiarism".

11.4 Predatory Journals

Predatory magazines are publishers or magazines that do not actually exist. Although they resemble real journals and appear to be serious, they are not. What these journals have in common is that they are all Open Access and charge authors a fee per publication, without the intention of providing the services expected, such as peer review [1, 2, 4].

Charging per publications is a legitimate business model, however, and there are serious, prestigious journals that charge authors per publication. Therefore, charging does not necessarily make the journal predatory. There are journals that charge an APC according to their commercial model, but there is a whole process of peer review and their compliance with ethical objectives is ensured, etc. There are other journals which have a hybrid model. Normally, they are by subscription and do not charge authors for publication, but they are not open access. If the authors pay an APC, a sum, this journal then makes the article open to everyone and anybody can access the manuscript, read it, and download it.

The predatory journal is one that is going to charge a fee without any intention of providing services in return. In many cases, once the authors realize that they have submitted their article to a predatory journal, they are charged a fee to remove it.

11.4.1 How to Identify Predatory Journals

Identifying predatory journals is essential to maintaining academic integrity and research quality. New journals emerge daily that may seem legitimate, but in reality, they do not meet the minimum standards.

The "Think, Check, Submit" resource is very useful for authors seeking to evaluate the legitimacy of a journal, as it offers tools and guidance on how to discern between predatory and non-predatory publications [4]. On this site, there are a series of resources that authors can use to identify where to send book proposals or chapters for a book. This site is a campaign that was organized to ensure that minimum standards of peer review and publication ethics are met [4]. Another site to identify predatory journals is Beall's list (https://beallslist.net/), which identifies potential predatory open-access publishers.

Several techniques can be used to check whether a journal is predatory or serious [1, 2, 4]. To identify them, it is important to pay attention to certain characteristics:

- Predatory journals often use names that resemble a legitimate, reputable publication. Some of these journals may have an International Standard Serial Number (ISSN), but this may not be a legitimate identifier. They may even include fraudulent logos, such as that of PubMed or the Open Access Journals directory, despite not being associated with them.
- Sometimes, predatory journals may include impact factors that are unofficial or calculated in an unorthodox way.
- They often fail to provide clear information about the editorial board or responsible publisher. If there is an editorial board, it is made up of those who do not specialize in the journal's subject, for example, in dentistry.
- It should also stand out if they ask to send the manuscript as an email, that is, as an attached file, instead of establishing an online system for uploading sections of the manuscript, as serious journals do. These journals are very strict with the format of the manuscripts and submission procedures. Predatory journals usually have a "send it like it is", in any format, in which there are no suggestions or guidelines to authors. This should draw attention, as generally journals have a format which must be followed rigorously.
- Another warning sign is that these journals welcome submissions on a wide variety of topics, which may not be aligned with the journal's name or editorial focus. For example, these journals often invite dentists to submit articles from completely unrelated areas, such as finance, architecture, or archaeology, without any relationship to the experience or expertise of the researcher. Serious journals generally have a clear thematic focus.

- Additionally, they send messages appealing to the ego of the authors, suggesting that they need more submissions to complete the next upcoming issue or volume of the journal. This is a suspicious indicator, since prestigious journals generally do not have an issue with the number of article submissions. Of course, submission implies a cost for the authors since their business model is based on charging article processing fees (APC). However, the costs are usually unclear, some indicate not charging for publication, but instead say that they charge for the DOI, which in reality has a very low cost.
- Likewise, they promise to accept any type of work, with the advantage that the publication process will be fast. This publication speed is another warning, as serious journals typically have a thorough review process that can take 2–3 months [9], while those that promise a quick review often do not include a proper peer-review process.
- When reviewing articles published in predatory journals, it is common to find works that lack coherence or do not contribute to scientific knowledge [8]. The quality of these articles is frequently compromised by spelling and grammatical errors or inadequate data analysis, suggesting that not enough effort was invested in editorial review.
- Predatory journals might ask authors to send the manuscript ready to be published, not only in terms of format, also sections, references, etc. Therefore, the journal has not invested in galley proofs. As a result, spelling mistakes may occur. Of course, it is always possible for some spelling mistakes to happen, as both authors and proofreaders dedicated to making corrections might inadvertently overlook them [6]. However, if the manuscript is riddled with misspellings or poor grammar, it might be because it was published exactly as the authors submitted it.
- Finally, it is essential to consult the journal's policies regarding peer review and copyright. Some journals require that copyright be transferred to the publication, which should be clearly outlined in the author guidelines.

11.5 Predatory Conferences

Apart from predatory journals there are also predatory conferences, which they invite researchers and academics to submit abstracts, and even full manuscripts, to be published as conference proceedings. In other cases, they invite researchers to be keynote speakers or to host a session.

Ultimately, it might not amount to more than the cost of registration for the congress, but the benefit of going to a conference with prestigious researchers and scholars is the possibility of interacting with authors that you have studied, cited, and read. Therefore, those who attend benefit from establishing contact with those people. The editors of journals will be there, and it is worthwhile getting to know them. By attending these types of conferences, researchers and academic obtain a benefit just by being there and meeting other people.

However, this is not the case with predatory conferences. In conclusion, you must exercise caution with the target journal but also be careful with conference invitation.

11.6 Suggestions on How to Choose a Journal

There are sites that can help not only to identify predatory journals, but also aid with suggestions of alternative journals:

- Elsevier Journal Finder
- EndNote Match: Find the Best Fit Journals for Your Manuscript
- Journal/Author Name Estimator (JANE)
- Publish or Flourish Open Access
- Springer Journal Suggester
- Think. Check. Submit
- Web of Science Master List

Some are publishing houses, for example, Springer and Elsevier. These publishing houses have a series of magazines. For example, BMC-Oral Health is part of Springer-Nature. Journals that are not part of that conglomerate will not appear in their master lists. Journal Author Name Estimator (JANE) (http://jane.biosemantics.org) is another good site recommended by Think. Check. Submit. If you are yet to find a target journal for publication, you can use one of these resources.

11.7 Sending the Manuscript for Review

Once the right journal has been identified based on what has been discussed in this chapter, or based on your personal experience, you will enter the next stage of publication. Once the manuscript is submitted, it will first be reviewed by an administrative officer, that is, not by the editor but by someone who will verify that it is in the appropriate format, that the references are in the correct style, that the authors belong to their corresponding affiliation, that the keywords are identified, etc. In other words, it is not a review of the content but of format.

Plagiarism checks are also included as part of the manuscript review process. There is software specifically designed for this purpose, such as Turnitin® and iThenticate®, among other options available on the market. These programs assist in identifying overlapping similarities between the submitted manuscript and other publications, ensuring the originality of the content and upholding academic integrity.

Another issue to consider is self-plagiarism, which occurs when authors repeat their previously published content within their own work. This can happen due to duplications in methodology or by presenting the same results in two different articles. While it is not permissible to publish the same information twice, authors are allowed to use portions of information that has been previously published in another article. However, to do this it is essential to verify who holds the copyrights to that section of the results. By ensuring proper citation and adherence to copyright requirements, authors can avoid self-plagiarism while still building upon their previous work.

This stage can only be successfully completed after carefully reviewing the instructions to the authors, because the manuscript will be returned by secretariat, that is, it will not even go to peer review, if the authors do not meet these administrative requirements. Of course, this does not mean the manuscript was rejected, but revision is required because something was missing. The corresponding author, for example, or their affiliation. Ultimately, this will delay the process and be frustrating for the authors.

11.7.1 Editor Review

Once the article meets all the requirements of submission type, form and format, it goes to the editor. The editor will make a preliminary evaluation of whether the article should go to peer review, because as mentioned, peer-reviewers are volunteers, and they are giving up their time to review the article. Therefore, an editor will not submit an article for peer review if they do not think the quality is high enough to go to the reviewers. Again, there is no assurance of acceptance since a reviewer can still reject it. However, if the initial quality of the article is not sufficient or the topic doesn't correspond to the journal, the editor will reject it straight away.

At this stage, the editors can reject the manuscript for several reasons. For example, they might decide that the information is unreliable, that the research contains errors, or there is evidence of data fabrication. Additionally, they might identify examples of plagiarism, find that the data has been previously published or that the research does not adhere to established ethical procedures.

In addition to the authority to reject manuscripts, editors can also retract published articles. This occurs when a manuscript that has been published in a journal later comes to light as including previously published material, data that does not belong to the authors, or another significant issue that calls the integrity of the work into question. There is a registry available for authors whose publications have been retracted, which can be found at: https://www.enago.com/academy/database-of-retracted-papers-launched-for-researchers/ [10].

A review conducted by Rapani et al. [11] of retracted articles in the dental literature found that the primary reason for retraction was research misconduct. This misconduct was frequently related to plagiarism, but also included issues such as unreliable data and duplication or fabrication of results. Additionally, the study identified scientific errors, particularly flaws in methodology, as contributing factors for retraction [11].

Editors may retract published papers for various other reasons, including double publication, unpaid publication charges, compromised peer-review processes (where the review was not transparent), and copyright violation, among others.

Another issue is self-plagiarism, which occurs when authors repeat themselves. This might be due to duplications in methodology, but can also involve presenting the same results in two different articles. As mentioned, it is not permitted to publish the same information twice, but you can use portions of information that has been published in another article. To do so, you must identify who holds the rights to that section of the results. This rule generally does not apply to conference presentations. As such, you can convert a conference presentation into a publication. However, this manuscript should be published after the paper was presented in a conference.

11.7.2 Peer Review

If a manuscript is well written and the journal was appropriately selected, it will go to a peer-review panel who will give their verdict. Reviewers have four options: accept it, minor revisions, major revisions or rejection. Then, with the verdict it goes back to the editor and the editor decides whether to continue the process or not according to the suggestions or evaluation of the reviewers and their own evaluation. The editor can reject the manuscript or request revisions, in which case a new peer review is commenced until it is finally rejected or accepted. Figure 11.1 is a simplified diagram illustrating the process of submitting a manuscript to a journal, outlining the key steps in a sequential manner.

Furthermore, it is essential for researchers to recognize the importance of persistence in the publication process. Rejection is a common experience in academic publishing, and it should not be viewed as a reflection of the quality of the research. Instead, develop an "elephant hide" and do not be discouraged by criticism, feedback, and rejections from editors or reviewers. As mentioned, 50% of the manuscripts that JDR receives are rejected and do not go through review. Researchers

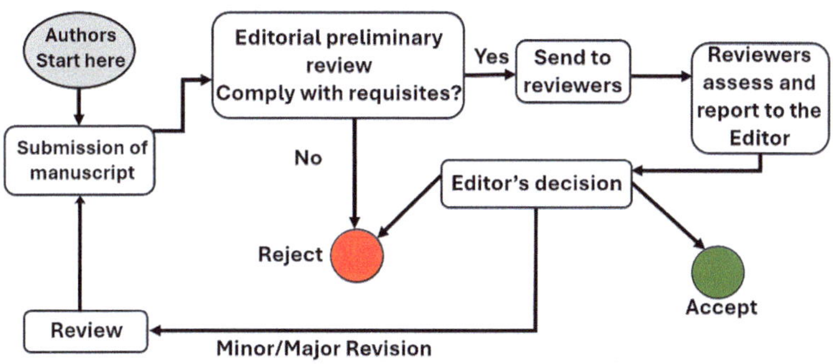

Fig. 11.1 Simplified diagram of submission of a manuscript through the journal's submission system

should approach a rejection as an opportunity for growth and improvement. By carefully considering the feedback provided by reviewers and making necessary revisions, researchers can enhance their work and increase their chances of acceptance in subsequent submissions.

This whole process may take at least 2 or 3 months [9]. Normally, article review is done by peer-reviewers who volunteer their time and do not receive payment, but a serious review can take two or three hours. This is why it is very important that you do not send it to multiple journals at a time. It is also important for an editor to decide whether to send it to reviewers. Therefore, we should assume the responsibility of preparing our manuscript to make it as easy as possible for an editor to send the manuscript for peer review.

11.8 Final Remarks

This chapter emphasized the importance of overcoming the barriers associated with research publication and highlighted key considerations in the selection of an appropriate journal for dissemination of the research. Through carefully selecting the appropriate journal, navigating the administrative requirements of submission, and remaining resilient in the face of potential setbacks, researchers can successfully share their findings with peers and the broader community. Ultimately, publication not only validates the efforts of researchers but also enriches collective understanding of complex issues and drives progress across various fields of inquiry. As we continue to navigate the evolving landscape of academic publishing, it is imperative that researchers remain committed to the principles of transparency, rigour, and ethical responsibility, ensuring that their contributions are recognized and valued.

References

1. Zettel C. How to select a journal for publication: a comprehensive guide for researchers. 2022. https://www.aje.com/arc/how-to-choose-a-journal-for-publication/. Accessed 10 Oct 2024.
2. PLOS. How to choose the journal that's right for your study. 2024. https://plos.org/resource/how-to-choose-journal/. Accessed 10 Oct 2024.
3. Wiley. How to choose a journal for publication. 2024. https://www.wiley.com/en-us/network/publishing/research-publishing/forward-series/how-to-choose-a-journal-for-publication-journal-finder-tool. Accessed 10 Oct 2024.
4. Think. Check. Submit. 2024. https://thinkchecksubmit.org/. Accessed 10 Oct 2024.
5. Springer Nature. How to choose a target journal. 2023. https://www.springer.com/gp/authors-editors/journal-author/how-to-choose-a-target-journal/1396. Accessed 10 Oct 2024.
6. Taylor R. Medical writing: a guide for clinicians, educators, and researchers. 1st ed. New York: Springer; 2018.
7. Eaton KA, Holland GR, Giannobile WV, Hancocks S, Robinson PG, Lynch CD. How is research publishing going to progress in the next 20 years? Transcription of session for editors, associate editors, publishers and others with an interest in scientific publishing held at IADR

meeting in Seattle on Wednesday, 20 March 2013. Eur J Dent Educ. 2014;18:e25–33. https://doi.org/10.1111/eje.12089.

8. Nieminen P, Uribe SE. The quality of statistical reporting and data presentation in predatory dental journals was lower than in non-predatory journals. Entropy (Basel). 2021;16(23):468. https://doi.org/10.3390/e23040468.
9. Van Meerbeek B, Frankenberger R. How to "sell" your paper to a peer-reviewed journal. J Adhes Dent. 2016;18:95–6. https://doi.org/10.3290/j.jad.a35977.
10. Enago Academy. Database of retracted papers launched for researchers. 2022. https://www.enago.com/academy/database-of-retracted-papers-launched-for-researchers/. Accessed 10 Oct 2024.
11. Rapani A, Lombardi T, Berton F, Del Lupo V, Di Lenarda R, Stacchi C. Retracted publications and their citation in dental literature: a systematic review. Clin Exp Dent Res. 2020;6:383–90. https://doi.org/10.1002/cre2.292.

Chapter 12
A Guide to Successful Conference Presentations

Sergio E. Uribe

12.1 Introduction

Communicating scientific results in conferences offer a valuable opportunity to present your findings, either final or preliminary, gather feedback and diverse opinions to refine your work, and, importantly, to build networks with colleagues and like-minded researchers. Poster presentations. This modality of making your work public plays a critical role in facilitating networking and interactions.

Poster presentations are gaining more acceptability these days. They allow a unique mix of visual and verbal communication. Posters allow researchers to engage in direct, one-to-one, conversation with a diverse audience, promoting discussion and collaboration. A poster serves as an effective communication tool for results and encourages dialogue among researchers with constructive feedback that enhances their work. Poster presentations are an opportunity for early-career researchers to gain confidence and presentation skills, including as distilling complex ideas and improving communication.

As research communication changes, the poster presentation format will continue to be essential for facilitating collaborations and increasing the visibility of scientific contributions. This chapter focuses on one of the most common and accessible formats for sharing scientific information: the poster presentation.

S. E. Uribe (✉)
Department of Conservative Dentistry and Oral Health, Riga Stradins University, Riga, Latvia

Department of Conservative Dentistry, Periodontology and Digital Dentistry, LMU University Hospital, LMU Munich, Germany
e-mail: sergio.uribe@rsu.lv

R. Mariño et al. (eds.), *Scientific Writing and Publication Strategies for Oral Health Professionals*, https://doi.org/10.1007/978-3-031-97916-3_12

12.2 Importance of Poster Presentations in Scientific Conferences

Conference presentations are an integral part of the scientific process. They provide researchers opportunities to share their findings, discuss and receive feedback, gain insights into the work of others, and build valuable professional networks. Figure 12.1 shows a view of a scientific poster session at a dental conference, illustrating the scale and diversity of ongoing research discussions. The presentation of research results provides an opportunity for networking, getting direct feedback, and refining research questions or approaches based on peer input. In addition, conference presentations are a testing ground for emerging scientists to develop their communication skills and gain visibility in their research field, often attracting potential collaborators, mentors, and funding opportunities. Through these interactions, conference presentations contribute to advancement and dissemination of knowledge. Here are some strategies to maximize your next presentation.

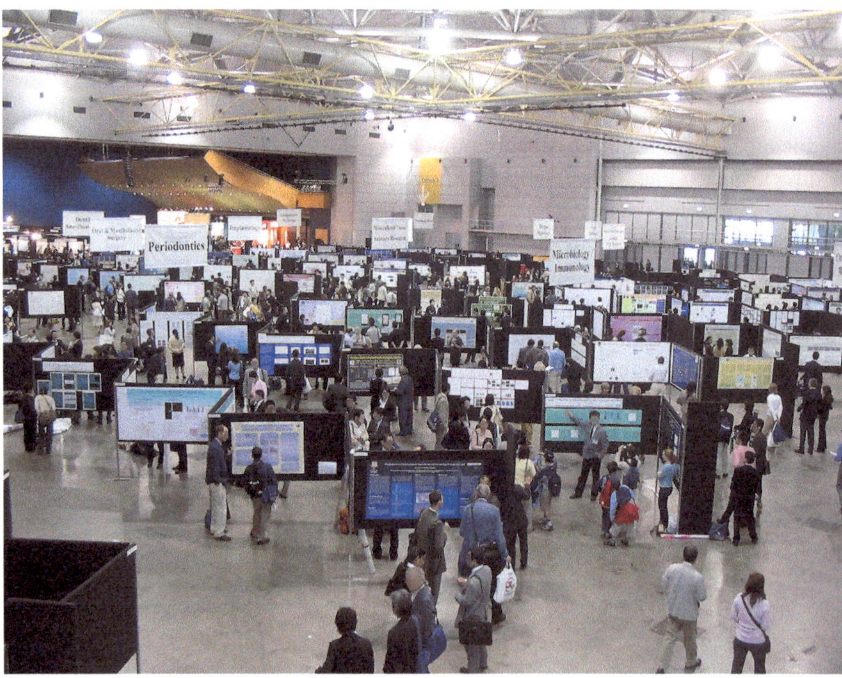

Fig. 12.1 Overview of poster presentations in dental conferences (source: Uribe, S. (2007, July 5). IADR Congress, Brisbane AU, 2007 [Photograph]. Flickr. https://flickr.com/photos/suribe/721458703/in/album-72157623646483678/, License: CC BY-SA 2.0)

12.3 Preparing for the Conference: Key Questions to Consider

Before attending a scientific conference to present your results, consider three basic questions to ensure that your presentation suits the audience and conference topics well.

1. **Why present this work?** Assess the significance of your research and its relevance to the field. Understanding why your work is important lays the foundation for a compelling presentation.
2. **Who is interested?** Determine the potential audience for your poster. Knowing who will be interested in your research will help you tailor your presentation to meet their expectations and interests.
3. **What are the most interesting aspects of my work?** Highlight the key points that capture the essence and novelty of your research. Focusing on these aspects will ensure that your presentation grabs attention and effectively engages the audience.

12.4 Presentation Formats

These are the basic formats for delivering a poster presentation at a scientific meeting:

1. **Open Poster Session:** This format allows for informal interactions. Attendees can approach the poster at their convenience and presenters can engage with viewers in a conversational manner.
2. **Dedicated Poster Symposium:** In this format, presenters typically give a brief synopsis of their work to a focused audience, often followed by discussions.
3. **Oral Presentation:** This involves presenting the research in a more formal setting, often with a set time limit for the presentation, followed by a question-and-answer session.
4. **Mixed Session:** This hybrid format incorporates both poster and oral elements. Presenters are assigned specific times to stand by their posters for a direct interaction, usually 3–5 min, ensuring dedicated audience engagement. Presenters participate in a formal oral presentation after the poster session, providing a more comprehensive overview of their research. This structured combination allows for detailed initial discussions at the poster, complemented by broader dissemination and formal Q&A during the subsequent oral session.

In this chapter, we will focus on poster presentations.

12.4.1 *The Poster Presentation*

A poster presentation represents an intermediate stage in your research process and, ideally, leads to the eventual publication of your results in a peer-reviewed journal. It is essential to carefully review the session guidelines, such as poster dimensions and designated times for standing by your poster. During the presentation, it can be helpful to ask a colleague to note down audience questions. View this as an opportunity to have experts review your work, identify any weaknesses, and provide feedback that can strengthen your research.

12.4.1.1 What Should Be in the Poster?

The poster is primarily a visual communication tool designed to succinctly and effectively convey the essence of your research through graphics rather than text. Figure 12.2 provides an example of a scientific poster display, highlighting the typical layout and visual emphasis used in research presentations. It should be a visual aid that enhances audience understanding of your study's purpose, methodology, and findings. A useful guideline to remember is that the poster should contain fewer words than the abstract of your paper, focusing more on diagrams, charts, and images to capture and retain viewer interest. A visually rich presentation draws attention and facilitates a clearer and quicker comprehension of the research conducted.

Important Before preparing your presentation, consult the official conference website for detailed and up-to-date requirements. These may include poster dimensions, file formats, time slots, and setup instructions. Following these ensures your work is correctly displayed and avoids last-minute issues. You can find examples of presentation guidelines, such as those for the International Association for Dental Research, here: https://bit.ly/iadr-guidelines.

Regardless of the format, effective presentations share key elements. The following are essential for any scientific poster:

1. **Title**: The title should be brief yet descriptive, concisely capturing the essence of your research. It should draw attendees' interest and give them a clear idea of the scientific issue you are addressing.
2. **Authors and Affiliation:** List all authors involved in the research, highlighting the presenting author. Include affiliations for each author and provide the presenter's email address to facilitate further communication.
3. **Introduction**: This section should set the stage for your research by explaining why your work is important and worth the audience's attention. Ensure to highlight the context and significance of your research.

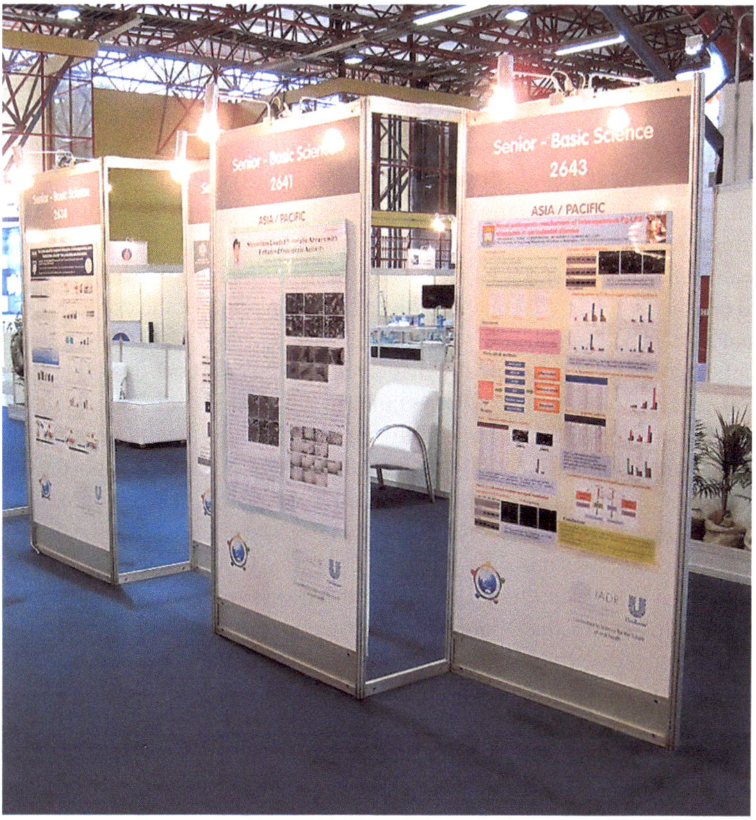

Fig. 12.2 Poster presentation (source: Uribe, S. (2012, July 6). IADR 2012 Iguazu [photograph]. Flickr. https://flickr.com/photos/suribe/7513202026/, License: CC BY-SA 2.0)

4. **Research Objective and Question:** Clearly state the objective or hypothesis and clarify the direction and purpose of your study.
5. **Materials and Methods:** Describe how the research was conducted. Include a diagram, if possible, to visually represent the experimental design or methodology, making it easier for viewers to understand the process you followed.
6. **Results**: Present what you have discovered through your research. Use figures, images, and graphs to convey your findings visually. Tables can supplement your visuals, providing detailed data in a structured format. Text should be used sparingly, mainly to emphasize key points and findings.
7. **Conclusion**: Summarize the insights gained from your research and answer the initial research question. This section should clearly state the implications of your findings and their relevance to the field.

12.4.1.2 Poster Design

Designing a scientific poster effectively is partly a matter of personal aesthetic preference, yet key principles help make a poster both compelling and informative. Figures 12.3 and 12.4 present a visual example that illustrates how an attractive poster should look. If using software such as PowerPoint, set the canvas or page size to the final print dimensions immediately. Avoid designing at standard slide size and enlarging later.

Please note that Figs. 12.3 and 12.4 may state "plain English." However, this should be considered in the context of the official language of the conference, which may not always be English.

Conference posters are typically displayed in either vertical or horizontal orientation, depending on the event. Always confirm the format in advance. It is generally preferable for your poster to be slightly smaller than the maximum board dimensions rather than risk it exceeding the available space. A successful poster typically features many graphical elements rather than text, regardless of orientation. These graphics, whether diagrams, charts, or images, should succinctly convey your research's core findings and data [2].

The text on the poster should be minimal but essential, designed to support the visual elements rather than dominate them. Any text included should be legible from 1 to 1.5 m away, ensuring viewers can easily read and understand the key messages without standing too close.

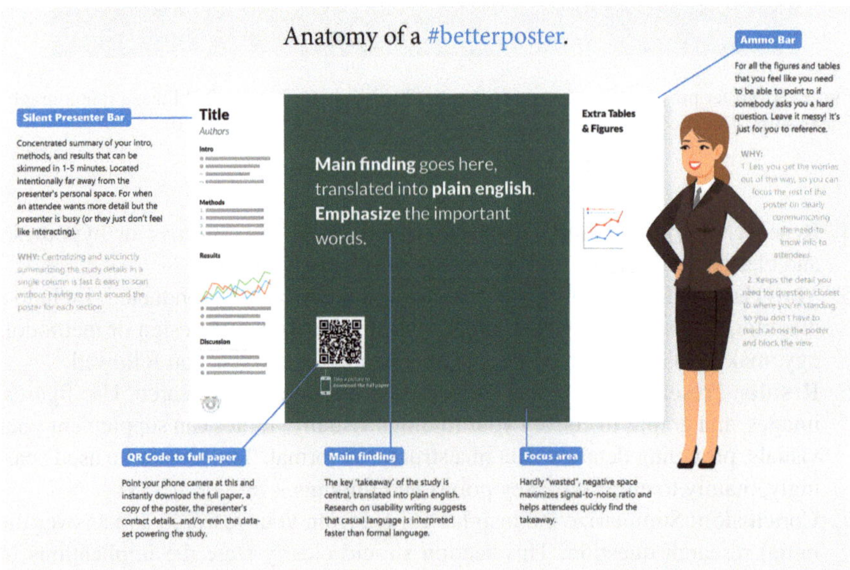

Fig. 12.3 Anatomy of a better poster—key elements for effective scientific communication [1] (source: Morrison M. Better scientific poster. Mike Morrison. 2019. https://osf.io/ef53g/, published under the terms of CC0 public domain)

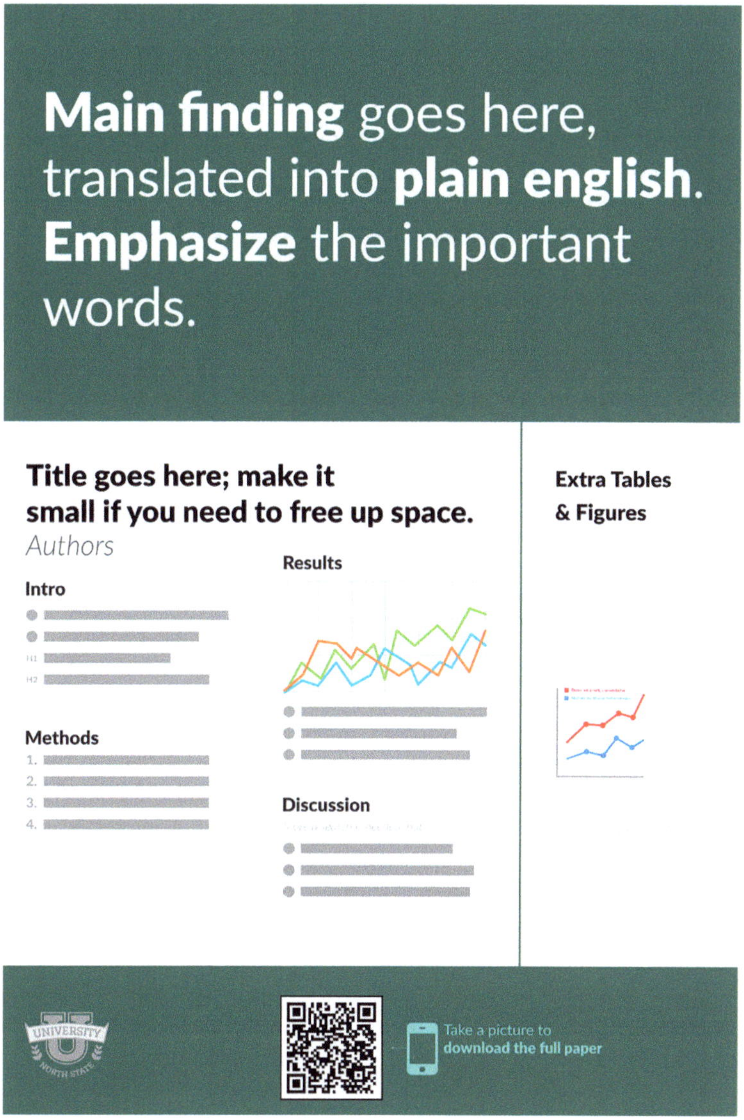

Fig. 12.4 Simplified poster layout for clear scientific communication [1] (source: Morrison M. Better scientific poster. Mike Morrison. 2019. https://osf.io/ef53g/, published under the terms of CC0 public domain)

For a professional and accessible presentation:

- **Font Size**: Use a **minimum font size of 24 points** for body text and at least **85 points for the main finding** to ensure visibility from a distance. The title and key messages should be bold and prominent. Any text included should be legible from 1 to 1.5 m away, ensuring viewers can easily read and understand the key messages without standing too close. This distance consideration is crucial in a busy conference setting, where space and viewer attention are limited.

- **Font Choice**: Select a clean, sans-serif font, such as **Arial**, **Helvetica**, or **Calibri**, for clarity. Avoid decorative fonts, as they can reduce readability.
- **Color Contrast**: Ensure high contrast between the text and background colors (e.g., dark text on a light background or vice versa) to enhance legibility.
- **Main Finding Emphasis**: Center and highlight the main finding in large, plain language, avoiding jargon to communicate the core message quickly.
- **Testing Readability**: Remember that what appears legible on a computer monitor may look different when printed on a large-scale poster. Print a test version of a section of the poster at full scale to check readability and layout.
- **QR Code for Full Paper**: Include a QR code linking to your paper, data, or additional content. Ensure your contact information (e.g., email) is clearly visible to enable follow-up communication.

Remember, a well-designed poster is not just a summary of your research. It is an invitation to engage with your work and a tool to facilitate discussion and networking with peers in your field [3].

Before final printing, generate an A4-size printout of the poster to check font size, layout structure, spelling, and color harmony [4].

Below are two contrasting examples of my poster design evolution. My first international conference poster was text-heavy, essentially a manuscript on a board, which was visually overwhelming and hard to grasp quickly (Fig. 12.5).

Compare this to my next poster, some conferences later, in Fig. 12.6. This poster was accompanied by printed handouts containing additional details, like a traditional abstract, which I provided to anyone seeking more information. The primary goal of the poster was to capture the attention of potential interested parties by presenting the key aspects of my research: its significance, our methods, findings, conclusions, and contact information [5]. This approach allowed the poster to highlight the essential points, with in-depth details available through verbal discussion

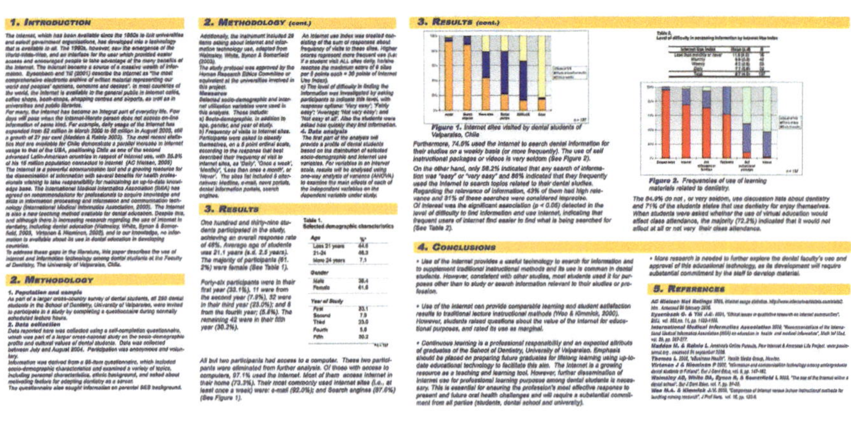

Fig. 12.5 Example of a poster with references

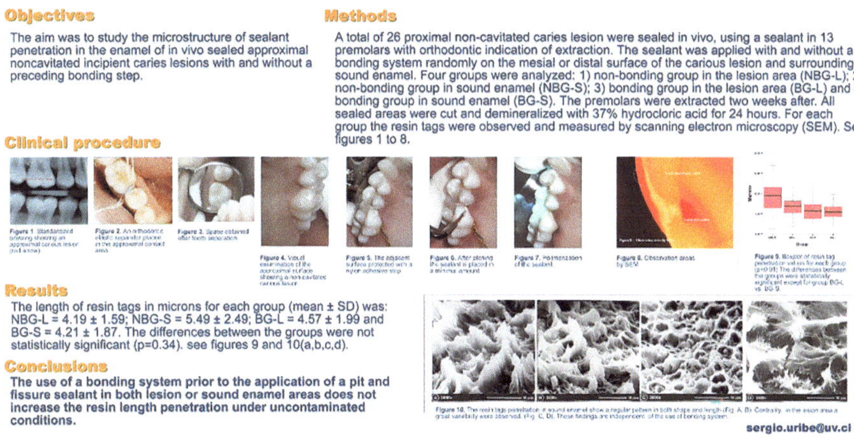

Fig. 12.6 Example of a poster without references

and supplementary handouts. This shift emphasized clarity and visual impact, making complex information accessible and engaging. It illustrates how effective poster design can enhance scientific communication at major conferences.

Even if you can see the references in my posters, I recommend that you do not add any references to the poster, or if you do, that you add them in the smallest font possible.

12.5 Additional Tips for Poster Presentations

1. Bring concise printed handouts or summary versions of your poster. These can be offered to attendees for later reference.
2. Include a QR code with a pdf of your poster to download and contact information.
3. Ensure to use a color-blind friendly palette; in general, avoid red, especially when combined with green [4].
4. Avoid the use of pie charts: They waste space and often lack precision. Pie charts make it difficult for viewers to interpret data accurately, especially with close values or numerous categories. Alternatives like bar charts or tables offer clearer, more direct comparisons and are better suited for quickly conveying information on posters, where visual clarity and space are essential.
5. Add a picture of the presenter: Add a small presenter photo to the poster so viewers can easily identify you during the session.
6. If you need to present using a computer, it would be ideal to access the room beforehand to check the setup—ensuring colors, size, and display look right, especially if using a computer that is not your own.

7. It doesn't matter if you use less time than assigned, but it is unacceptable to exceed it. In international conferences, you will be cut off when your time is up, so make sure to manage your time effectively.
8. Although basic materials are usually provided, carry your own pins or adhesive tape as a precaution.

12.6 Common Errors

Creating a compelling scientific poster involves much more than simply presenting data; it is about communicating your message effectively to interested researchers. A poster is not meant to be overly decorative or entertaining, but thoughtful design plays a crucial role in conveying information in a clear and engaging manner [5, 6]. If you feel that extensive details are essential, a preprint may be a better medium to provide in-depth content. Here are some common design missteps to avoid in poster presentations:

1. **Misalignment**: Disjointed visual elements where different parts of the poster do not line up can make your poster look disorganized and difficult to follow.
2. **Overuse of Text**: Large blocks of text can overwhelm viewers. Posters should use concise language and bullet points to communicate key points quickly.
3. **Poor Color Choices**: Using more than five colors can make a poster appear chaotic and distract from the content. Similarly, gradient fills in colored boxes may appear unprofessional or distract from the text.
4. **Inappropriate Fonts and Text Features**: Utilizing more than three typefaces or fonts like Comic Sans can make a poster seem less serious or harder to read. Over-stylized text features such as TEXT IN ALL CAPS, underlined text, or text with shadows can strain readability.
5. **Inadequate Graphical Representations**: Unlabeled error bars in graphs, 3-D graphs that clutter rather than clarify, and pixelated images detract from the poster's scientific credibility.
6. **Spacing Issues**: A lack of free space or too many visual elements can make a poster feel cluttered and make it difficult for viewers to absorb the information easily.
7. **Preparing a Poster in the Wrong Orientation:** Always confirm the format in advance. It is generally preferable for your poster to be slightly smaller than the maximum board dimensions.

12.7 After the Poster Presentation: Next Steps

12.7.1 Networking Opportunities

Once the session ends, follow up with new contacts. A brief thank-you email can help establish ongoing communication. You may also connect with participants via platforms like LinkedIn to stay informed about their work.

12.7.2 Prepare the Paper

Use the feedback gathered during your presentation to refine your manuscript before submission. A poster session is often a pre-publication checkpoint, not the final output.

Key takeaways

- **Preparation and Clarity**: Ensure your poster presents essential information succinctly and legibly, using minimal text and focusing instead on graphics to communicate key findings. Always consider the viewer's perspective: what they need to know, how they will interpret visuals and how accessible the information is from a distance
- **Guidelines Compliance**: Carefully review conference guidelines on poster size, layout, and time allocations. Adhering to these guidelines not only demonstrates professionalism but also enhances the impact of your presentation
- **Engagement and Feedback**: Use the poster session as an opportunity to interact with experts, gather feedback, and refine your research. Responding to questions and critiques with openness allows for valuable insights that can strengthen your study before publication
- **Networking**: Conference presentations are as much about building connections as they are about sharing findings. Be prepared with contact information and additional materials, such as printed handouts or QR codes, to facilitate follow-up conversations and future collaboration

12.8 Conclusion

In this chapter, we have discussed the importance of conference presentations as a dynamic and interactive component of scientific communication. Conference presentations are vital for disseminating research, gathering valuable feedback, and building connections within the scientific community [7]. This chapter provided practical insights into preparing and delivering effective poster presentations.

Effective poster presentations require thoughtful design, clear messaging, and adherence to best practices in visual communication—prioritizing simplicity, readability, and strategic use of space to enhance viewer engagement.

Key takeaways include focusing on clarity and minimal text, following conference guidelines, and designing with readability in mind. By making the most of this interactive format, researchers can refine their work, engage meaningfully with peers, and enhance the impact of their research. Effective conference presentations serve as a foundation for future publication, ensuring a broader reach and a stronger network of professional support.

References

1. Morrison M. Better scientific poster. 2019. https://osf.io/ef53g/. Accessed 10 Oct 2024.
2. Faulkes Z. Better posters: plan, design and present an academic poster. Exeter, England: Pelagic; 2021. https://pelagicpublishing.com/products/better-posters-zen-faulkes?srsltid=AfmBOooRrHe3T3urtvA5HDAjg-sGPx8oa0B2WvP-4ZsOU45WiNG_b9F3. Accessed 10 Oct 2024
3. Bourne PE. Ten simple rules for making good oral presentations. PLoS Comput Biol. 2007;3(4):e77. https://doi.org/10.1371/journal.pcbi.0030077.
4. Katsnelson A. Colour me better: fixing figures for colour blindness. Nature. 2021;598(7879):224–5. https://doi.org/10.1038/d41586-021-02696-z.
5. Jambor H, et al. Creating clear and informative image-based figures for scientific publications. PLoS Biol. 2021;19:1–25. https://doi.org/10.1371/journal.pbio.3001161.
6. Gemayel R. How to design an outstanding poster. FEBS J. 2018;285:1180–4. https://doi.org/10.1111/febs.14420.
7. Miller JE. Preparing and presenting effective research posters. Health Serv Res. 2007;42:311–28. https://doi.org/10.1111/j.1475-6773.2006.00588.x.

Chapter 13
Navigating the Peer-Review Process

Sergio E. Uribe

13.1 Introduction

Peer review is a fundamental part of scientific publishing, a process by which experts in the field evaluate the quality, validity, and originality of research before publication. This review mechanism ensures that only high-quality research is published, thereby maintaining the integrity of the scientific literature [1].

This chapter provides a perspective on the peer-review process, highlighting its role in academic publishing by ensuring quality of research before publication. It explores the motivations, challenges, and expectations of both reviewers and editors, offering insights into how reviewers evaluate submissions based on validity, methodology, and relevance. The chapter emphasizes constructive feedback, enabling authors to improve their work through reviewer input. The chapter also provides strategies for effective reviewing, including objectivity, clear comments, and ethical practices. Authors receive practical advice on managing and responding to reviewers' comments, helping them to deal with critical feedback and prioritize revisions professionally.

The goal is to equip researchers with tools to navigate the peer-review process effectively and ethically [2].

S. E. Uribe (✉)
Department of Conservative Dentistry and Oral Health, Riga Stradins University, Riga, Latvia

Department of Conservative Dentistry, Periodontology and Digital Dentistry, LMU University Hospital, LMU Munich, Germany
e-mail: sergio.uribe@rsu.lv

R. Mariño et al. (eds.), *Scientific Writing and Publication Strategies for Oral Health Professionals*, https://doi.org/10.1007/978-3-031-97916-3_13

13.2 A Short History of Peer Review [3]

The term "peer review" emerged in the 1970s, but its roots can be traced back to the Royal Society of London's Philosophical Transactions, which began publication in 1665. Initially managed by the Society's secretaries, the process lacked clear standards. Formal implementation of expert referees began in 1832, although the practice had already been introduced abroad, particularly at the Académie des Sciences in Paris.

Historically, peer review was not always standard. Journals like *Annalen der Physik*, which published Einstein's groundbreaking papers, initially relied on editorial discretion. Anecdotal evidence tells us that even renowned scientists had issues with peer review. Albert Einstein, for instance, withdrew a paper on gravitational waves from *Physical Review*, citing disapproval of having his work shown to peers without his consent.

Modern peer review gained acceptance in the twentieth century with the growth of independent scientific journals. In 1973, the journal *Nature* made peer-review standard practice to prevent accusations of favoritism and elitism.

While peer review aims to guard against inaccurate claims and ensure the integrity of published work, its effectiveness has been debated. A 1998 review identified low reliability, lack of objective criteria, frequent errors, and bias against novel work. However, high-quality reviews can lead to more citations, positively impacting a work's reception. Frustrations with traditional peer review have led to alternative systems. Some journals, like *PLOS One*, have made the reviewing process more public, publishing "technically sound" research and allowing readers to judge its relevance. Others advocate for a "market of ideas" approach where readers identifies the best research.

13.3 Purpose of Peer Review [4]

The primary goals of peer review are to validate research findings, enhance the quality of published work, and maintain the credibility of academic journals.

Peer review serves as a filter for scientific journals. It is a fundamental self-regulation mechanism within the academic community, ensuring that published research meets established scientific standards, ideally allowing reproducibility (obtaining identical results reanalyzing the original data) and replicability (achieving consistent results collecting new data to test the same hypothesis using the same methods).

13.3.1 Who Are the Peer Reviewers?

Most scientific journals today are published by private companies. Some journals are affiliated with a professional or scientific society, which usually provides the editorial board and editor-in-chief to oversee the editorial process while the publisher handles the administrative side.

The editorial board is composed of experts in the field of the specific journal, and the editor uses their knowledge to find appropriate reviewers for the submitted papers.

13.3.2 What Do the Editors Do?

Editors in scientific journals have roles in publication, serving as intermediaries between authors, reviewers, and the scientific community. Scientific editors play a complex role that is essential to maintaining the quality and integrity of scientific publishing. They evaluate manuscripts for relevance, make the initial decision of whether to reject or send to peer review, manage the peer review process, and make final publication decisions based on feedback. Editors commission content, organize special issues, maintain ethical standards, manage conflicts of interest, and address misconduct. They engage with the research community by attending conferences, keeping on current trends. They build relationships to encourage submissions and collaborations.

13.4 The Peer-Review Process

Figure 13.1 illustrates the typical peer-review workflow, outlining each stage from manuscript submission by the author to editorial assessment, reviewer evaluation, and final publication.

The peer-review process usually involves the following steps (Fig 13.1):

1. **Submission**: The author submits their manuscript to a peer-reviewed journal. This initial step involves preparing and sending a complete manuscript that adheres to the journal's submission guidelines (Step 1).
2. **Editorial Assessment**: The editor initially screens the manuscript for its relevance and adherence to the journal's scope and quality standards. This step determines whether the manuscript should proceed to full peer review.
3. **Reviewer Assignment:** If the manuscript passes the initial screening, the editor identifies and invites appropriate peer reviewers who are experts in the manuscript's subject matter (Step 2).
4. **Peer Review:** The assigned reviewers thoroughly evaluate the manuscript, assessing its methodology, validity, and contribution to the field (Step 3). They provide detailed feedback and recommendations, such as accepting, revising, or rejecting (Step 4) [5].
5. **Editorial Decision:** Based on the reviewers' feedback, the editor decides (Step 5) on the manuscript's fate—whether it is accepted as is, needs minor or major revisions, should be resubmitted after major changes, or is rejected.

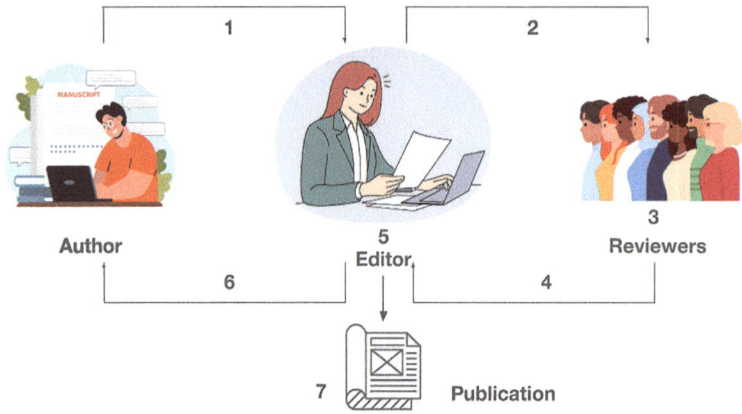

Fig. 13.1 The peer-review process (images by inspiring_team (for author); Vasilyeu (for editor); aprint22com (for reviewers); smoki (for publication)/YayImages.com)

6. **Author Notification:** The author is informed of the editorial decision and any reviewer feedback. If revisions are required, detailed comments are provided to guide these modifications (Step 6).
7. **Publication**: Once the manuscript meets all required standards and revisions, it is accepted for publication. The final step is for the manuscript to be formally published in the journal, contributing to the scientific body of knowledge in dental research (Step 7).

13.4.1 Types of Peer Review

There are several models of peer review, each with different advantages:

1. **Single-Anonymous Peer Review:** The reviewers know the authors' identities but not vice versa. This is common across many scientific and medical journals.
2. **Double-Blind Peer Review:** The identities of both the authors and reviewers are concealed, aiming to reduce bias related to the authors' reputations or institutional affiliations.
3. **Open Peer Review:** Both authors and reviewers are known to each other, and review comments are often published, enhancing transparency but possibly hindering candid feedback.
4. **Other Types of Peer Review:** Other types include *Triple-blind review*, which, although logistically complex, provides complete anonymity for unbiased evaluations. *Post-publication review* encourages ongoing critique but can lead to unmoderated debates. *Registered reports* undergo a two-stage review for methodological rigor and comprehensive documentation. *Collaborative review* promotes author-reviewer dialogue for improved feedback, although it is

time-consuming. *Portable review* increases efficiency by transferring reviews between journals, reducing redundancy, and accelerating publication for the benefit of the scientific community.

13.5 Common Reasons for Rejection

I recall attending a seminar by the then-editor of the Journal of Dental Research. He gave three pieces of advice to authors:

1. Read the instructions to authors,
2. Read the instructions to authors,
3. Read the instructions to authors.

Based on my experience, I would add some advice of my own to these three excellent tips:

- Ensure that your idea and the need for the research are both very well-founded. This means there should be a previous publication indicating the knowledge gap your research will fill.
- Follow the recommendations of the relevant EQUATOR NETWORK Guide. To determine the appropriate guide, visit https://www.goodreports.org/ [6].
- For quantitative research: unless you are statistician or have strong statistical background, consult a statistician or study design specialist **before** starting your study.

Table 13.1 summarizes the most common reasons dental scientific journals reject research manuscripts.

13.6 How to Reply to Reviewers [10]

After months (or years!) of completing your study, writing up the results and submitting to your chosen journal, you'll receive reviewer comments, and it is now time to revise. Establish a clear plan for your response in order to stay on track and ensure you don't overlook any necessary changes. It is essential to respond to **all** reviewer comments. For suggestions indicating missing elements, address these by adding the necessary information. However, if a reviewer requests a change you disagree with, clearly explain your reasoning for not implementing it.

Table 13.1 Most common reasons for rejecting research manuscripts [6–9]

Reason	Section	Examples	Check items
Lack of originality, novelty, or significance	Introduction	No reference to why this research needs to be done	Support the need of the new research by referencing a recent paper or review that identifies a gap in the knowledge your paper aims to address
Unclear research question	Introduction	The study question is not clearly structured or defined	Use a structured approach like PICO for clinical questions and clearly describe any hypotheses, such as: "*We hypothesize that intervention A will reduce the incidence of X by 15%.*"
Mismatch with the journal's aims and scope	Methods	Findings that are of interest to a very narrow audience not targeted by the journal	Review the main references in your paper; if they commonly cite the journal you are targeting, it likely aligns with the journal's scope
Flaws in study design	Methods	Poor experimental design with vague or inadequate methods	Register your protocol and adhere to relevant reporting guidelines like STROBE for observational studies or CONSORT for clinical trials [8] For quantitative studies: consult a statistician **before** starting the study
Erroneous or unsupported data interpretation or conclusions	Discussion	Conclusions are disproportionate to the results or are not supported by the study design	Considering your sample size, statistical assumptions, lack of multivariable analysis, confounders, and Hill's criteria, avoid using causality language if your study design does not aim to establish causality
Poor presentation	All	Missing section, lack of organization and illation, references	Review the journal's instructions for authors as you begin to prepare your submission and ask a co-author to review the manuscript for compliance with the instructions for authors before submitting

13.6.1 Stay Calm and Considerate

Occasionally, you may receive frustrating comments. While it might seem that reviewers need to spend more time considering your work, are overly critical, or lack the necessary experience, remember that a lot can get lost in translation. Always assume that reviewers have the best of intentions and reply accordingly [11].

The goal of peer-review comments is to verify and strengthen your work, ultimately making it a more effective expression of your study. Reviewers represent the general audience of the journal, and their reactions can help you create a better and clearer publication for your readers.

After reviewing the comments on your manuscript, it may be helpful to step back and clear your mind. When you return, ask yourself: what are the fundamental issues the reviewer wants you to address? Usually, you will find three types of comment. Some are trivial, addressing a typo or an evident mistake, and these are easy to address. The second type of comment is when the reviewer didn't understand something or got confused. This means it was our responsibility as writers for not being clear, and a correction is required to clarify the idea we wanted to express. The third type of comment occurs when the reviewer is not convinced by our results or interpretation. Addressing this usually requires us to provide additional information, such as a supplementary table with extra results. These comments require more time to address. In all cases, it is important to address the issue in the text itself, not only in the reply, but also by showing the reviewer that you have addressed their concern in the manuscript to ensure that future readers can benefit also.

13.6.2 Make a Plan for Revising and Responding

Do not lose sight of the important changes you want to make. Establishing a plan for revising and drafting your response to the reviewer can help you organize your steps, better understand what needs to be done and ensure a smoother process.

Checklist:

1. Be polite, grateful, and professional, even when you think a reviewer is wrong.
2. Avoid assuming a reviewer lacks expertise; they have taken the time to read your work thoroughly.
3. Respond fully to each reviewer's comment, leave no issue unaddressed.
4. Make it easy for the reviewer and editor to understand your response.
5. If you do not understand a review comment, it is okay to indicate this.
6. Provide supporting evidence for your statements and contentions.

13.6.3 Writing Your Response

Include a cover letter. Keep it brief but highlight important information about your changes and any points you want to clarify. If you found the reviewers' comments particularly useful, thank them for their thoughtful feedback.

Here's a short template to follow:

> Thank you for taking the time to review and comment on our manuscript, _____. The comments were constructive, and we have incorporated many suggestions into our revision…

(*continued*)

(continued)
All the changes are underlined (or highlighted)
We have responded to each comment individually below.
Reviewer 1. Comment 4.
Reviewer: Authors tend to mention about high caries risk, but no specific data given in terms of caries prevalence or severity cited
Reply: We have added the reference about the definition of caries risk, now it reads:
...and the prevalence of early childhood caries worldwide has been reported in 48% [12].
...and may increase caries risk, defined as having active cavitated or non-cavitated carious lesions among other signs or factors (AAPD, 2020) in primary teeth...

Assume that both the editor and the reviewers will see everything you write. Readers may also see your comments if you've submitted to a journal with an open peer-review process. Open review offers transparency and accountability, as both authors and reviewers are visible, fostering constructive feedback. However, it may discourage candid critiques and introduce potential bias if reviewers feel less anonymous.

Responses should be clear, non-emotional, and easy to understand. Respond inline to each comment, providing line numbers to indicate where the corresponding changes can be found.

Sample responses:

Write your response, take a break, and come back. Reread your comments and make sure they are calm and professional. If you're unsure what to say, use these examples of reviewer responses for inspiration. It is also important that all authors are aware of the reviewer comments and participate in the reply, **ensuring that all contributors agree with the final manuscript** before resubmission.

Reviewer 1 Comment: The increase from time a to time b would be clearer with a line plot with a 95% confidence interval.
Reply: Thank you very much. We have added a new figure; see Figure 4.
Reviewer 2 Comment: There is a repetition of ideas in the third paragraph of the discussion
Response: Thank you, we have removed the second sentence, now it reads: ....

13.6.4 Dealing with Conflicting Comments

It is almost inevitable that you will come across reviewers who disagree about a course of action, and even the editor may have a differing opinion from the reviewers. Here are some strategies for navigating these situations:

Reviewer vs. Editor Generally, the editor should be able to provide comments related to the journal's editorial policy and scope. If the editor disagrees with a suggested edit, cite the comments in your response to the reviewers.

Reviewer vs. Reviewer In situations where two reviewers provide conflicting advice, the editor can guide the journal's standards and suggest the most appropriate course of action. If not, you can write to the editor for guidance. As with the previous scenario, cite the editor's advice in your response.

In cases where an editor does not provide any specific direction, it falls upon the authors to decide based on the evidence at hand.

13.7 Criticisms and Challenges

Despite its widespread acceptance, peer review is not without criticism. Some argue that it can be slow, biased, or inconsistent and that inaccuracies can still occur in published articles even after peer review. For example, several Nobel Prize-winning papers were rejected the first time they were sent to a journal, such as Hans Krebs's paper on the citric acid cycle [13], which later won the 1953 Nobel Prize in Medicine, or Peter Ratcliffe's manuscript on how cells sense and adapt to oxygen availability [14], which later won the 2019 Nobel Prize in Medicine with Willian Kaelin and Gregg Semenza. More recently, Katalin Kariko and Drew Weissman's paper on nucleoside base modification that enables the development of effective mRNA vaccines was rejected not once but twice, and it finally won its authors the Nobel Prize in Medicine in 2023 [15].

In recent years, several initiatives have emerged to recognize and reward the contributions of peer reviewers. **Publons**, a platform dedicated to tracking and showcasing peer-review activities, initially ranked reviewers by country, field, and institution, offering visibility for their efforts. Later acquired by **Clarivate**, a company managing the **Web of Science** index—an influential database of scholarly citations—Publons integrated ORCID, a unique identifier for researchers. **ORCID** (Open Researcher and Contributor ID) provides a persistent digital identifier, linking researchers' work across publications, affiliations, and peer reviews. Now, each completed peer review can be automatically added to a reviewer's ORCID profile, formally recognizing and documenting their contributions.

Nevertheless, the consensus within the scientific community is that peer review remains the most effective method for ensuring scientific quality and integrity. Despite its imperfections, peer review is an essential component of scholarly communication. It offers a structured and systematic approach to evaluating research quality and promotes a culture of continuous improvement and innovation in scientific inquiry [16].

13.8 Conclusion

The peer-review process plays a vital role in maintaining the quality, integrity, and relevance of academic research. This chapter provided insights into the complex dynamics of peer review and highlighted its importance in refining research through constructive feedback from knowledgeable reviewers. The process not only ensures studies meet high methodological standards but promotes a collaborative environment for improving research.

Despite challenges such as bias and delays, peer review remains a cornerstone of scholarly communication. Reviewers, often volunteers, contribute to the advancement of science by providing detailed, objective critiques that help authors improve their manuscripts. For authors, responding effectively to reviewers' comments—by addressing concerns or providing rationale for alternative approaches—can strengthen both the research and its presentation.

References

1. Open Science Framework. https://osf.io/aynr5. Accessed 10 Oct 2024.
2. Peer reviewing research. https://www.equator-network.org/toolkits/peer-reviewing-research/. Accessed 10 Oct 2024.
3. History of philosophical transactions. 2024. https://royalsociety.org/journals/publishing-activities/publishing350/history-philosophical-transactions/. Accessed 10 Oct 2024.
4. Swartz MK. The importance of peer review. J Pediatr Health Care. 2008;22(6):333–4. https://doi.org/10.1016/j.pedhc.2008.08.004.
5. Baker M. 1,500 scientists lift the lid on reproducibility. Nature. 2016;533(7604):452–4. https://doi.org/10.1038/533452a.
6. Higgins J, Welch V. Cochrane handbook for systematic reviews of interventions. The Cochrane Collaboration. 2024. https://training.cochrane.org/handbook. Accessed 10 Oct 2024.
7. Streiner DL. A shortcut to rejection: how not to write the results section of a paper. Can J Psychiatry. 2007;52:385–9. https://doi.org/10.1177/070674370705200608.

8. Moher D, Liberati A, Tetzlaff J, Altman DG. Preferred reporting items for systematic reviews and meta-analyses: the PRISMA statement. PLoS Med. 2009;6(7):e1000097. https://doi.org/10.1371/journal.pmed.1000097.
9. Public Library of Science (PLoS). How to receive and respond to peer review feedback. 2020. https://plos.org/resource/how-to-receive-and-respond-to-peer-review-feedback/. Accessed 10 Oct 2024.
10. Williams HC. How to reply to referees' comments when submitting manuscripts for publication. J Am Acad Dermatol. 2004;51:79–83. https://doi.org/10.1016/j.jaad.2004.01.049.
11. Uribe SE, Innes N, Maldupa I. The global prevalence of early childhood caries: A systematic review with meta-analysis using the WHO diagnostic criteria. Int J Paediatr Dent. 2021;31:817–30. https://doi.org/10.1111/ipd.12783.
12. De La Garza H, Vashi NA. The role of peer review in the scientific process. In: Faintuch J, Faintuch S, editors. Integrity of scientific research. Cham: Springer; 2022. p. 409–16. https://doi.org/10.1007/978-3-030-99680-2_41.
13. Borrell B. Nature rejects Krebs's paper, 1937. The Scientist Magazine®. 2010. https://www.the-scientist.com/nature-rejects-krebss-paper-1937-43452. Accessed 10 Oct 2024.
14. Anorak News. https://www.anorak.co.uk/459485/news/sir-peter-j-ratcliffe-the-1992-rejection-letter-from-nature-for-the-paper-he-submitted-on-his-nobel-prize-winning-work.html. Accessed 10 Oct 2024.
15. Bansal A. From rejection to the Nobel Prize: Karikó and Weissman's pioneering work on mRNA vaccines, and the need for diversity and inclusion in translational immunology. Front Immunol. 2023;14. https://doi.org/10.3389/fimmu.2023.1306025.
16. Nosek BA, Alter G, Banks GC, Borsboom D, Bowman SD, Breckler SJ, et al. Scientific standards. Promoting an open research culture. Science (New York, NY). 2015;348(6242). https://doi.org/10.1126/science.aab2374.

Index

R. Mariño et al. (eds.), *Scientific Writing and Publication Strategies for Oral Health Professionals*, https://doi.org/10.1007/978-3-031-97916-3

MIX
Papier aus verantwortungsvollen Quellen
Paper from responsible sources
FSC® C105338

If you have any concerns about our products,
you can contact us on
ProductSafety@springernature.com

In case Publisher is established outside the EU,
the EU authorized representative is:
Springer Nature Customer Service Center GmbH
Europaplatz 3, 69115 Heidelberg, Germany

Printed by Libri Plureos GmbH
in Hamburg, Germany